INESCAPABLE DECISIONS

INESCAPABLE DECISIONS

The Imperatives
of Health Reform

David Mechanic

Transaction Publishers
New Brunswick (U.S.A.) and London (U.K.)

Copyright © 1994 by Transaction Publishers, New Brunswick, New Jersey 08903.

All rights reserved under International and Pan-American Copyright Conventions. No part of this book may be reproduced or transmitted in any form or by any means, electronic or mechanical, including photocopy, recording, or any information storage and retrieval system, without prior permission in writing from the publisher. All inquiries should be addressed to Transaction Publishers, Rutgers—The State University, New Brunswick, New Jersey 08903.

Library of Congress Catalog Number: 93-13425
ISBN: 1-56000-121-6
Printed in the United States of America

Library of Congress Cataloging-in-Publication Data
Mechanic, David, 1936-
  Inescapable decisions : the imperatives of health reform / David Mechanic.
    p. cm.
  Essays adapted from previously published materials.
  Includes bibliographical references and index.
  ISBN 1-56000-121-6 (cloth)
  1. Medical policy—United States. 2. Social medicine—United States. 3. Health planning—United States. I. Title.
  [DNLM: 1. Health Policy—United States—collected works. 2. Delivery of Health Care—organization & administration—United States—collected works. 4. United States.
WA 540 AA1 M4i 1993]
RA395.A3M418 1993
362.1'0973—dc20
DNLM/DLC
for Library of Congress
                                                    93-13425
                                                    CIP

For Kate

Contents

Acknowledgments

The essays in this book are adapted from previously published materials. Chapter 1, based on a paper entitled "The American Health Care System and Its Future" that appeared in March 1993 in *Medical Care Review*, is reprinted with the permission of the J.B. Lippincott Company. Chapter 2, "Sources of Countervailing Power in Medicine," appeared in the *Journal of Health Politics, Policy and Law*, copyright 1991 by Duke University Press and is reprinted with the permission of the publisher. Chapter 3, "Professional Judgment and the Rationing of Medical Care" (1992) is reprinted with the permission of the *Pennsylvania Law Review*. Chapter 4 includes segments that appeared in "Researching the Idea of Health" in *Social Psychiatry: Theory, Methodology, and Practice*, ed. P. Bebbington (New Brunswick, NJ:Transaction Publishers, 1991). Chapter 5 also includes sections published in "Promoting Health," *Society* (1990), copyright by Transaction Publishers. Chapter 6 is adapted from a 1989 article in *Pathways to Health*, eds. J. Bunker, D.S. Gomby and B.H. Kehrer, used with permission from the publisher, the Kaiser Family Foundation of Menlo Park, CA. Chapter 7 is reprinted from *Adolescents at Risk: Medical and Social Perspectives* (1992), edited by D. Rogers and E. Ginzberg, reprinted here by permission of Westview Press, Boulder, CO. Chapter 8 is based on two articles published with David Rochefort of Northeastern University that appeared in "Deinstitutionalization: An Appraisal of Reform," *Annual Review of Sociology* 16 (1990), and reprinted with permission of Annual Reviews, Inc., and "A Policy of Inclusion for the Mentally Ill" which appeared in *Health Affairs*. Chapter 9 is a revised paper from the *Annals of the American Academy of Political and Social Science* (1989) and is reproduced with the permission of Sage Publications. Chapter 10 includes some sections of a paper published in *Social Science and Medicine* 36, no. 2 (1993), reprinted with permission from Pergamon Press Ltd., Headington Hill Hall, Oxford, OX3 OBW, U.K. Appendix A was previously published in the *Journal of Health and Social Behavior*, a journal of the American Sociological Association. Appendix B appeared in *Health Affairs* 9 (1990). Special thanks are due to Kathryn Woods who helped on all aspects of preparation of this manuscript for publication. Her assistance is greatly appreciated.

Introduction

The American health care system is out of control. Despite varying efforts, costs continue to escalate with anticipated expenditures in 1992 of more than $800 billion. Growing numbers of persons are uninsured, and many more underinsured. The insurance market is in disarray, and individuals throughout the society feel increasingly insecure about their health coverage should they change jobs or lose their employment. Risk rating is practiced with a vengeance, and persons most in need of health insurance because of a serious illness or disability have difficulty acquiring insurance unless covered by large employer plans.

At the point of service delivery, there is much evidence that the high-technology interventionist type of medicine practiced in America has lost a sense of priorities and balance. Expensive and sometimes dangerous procedures of unknown efficacy are used promiscuously and often inappropriately while very basic preventive and primary care services are often unavailable, especially to disadvantaged populations greatly in need of basic services. Evidence is mounting of extraordinary waste while simple needs often go unattended. Incredibly complex administrative arrangements and heavy-handed regulations consume from a fifth to a quarter of the health care dollar.

Almost everyone agrees that our health system is in disarray and that major reform is needed. They disagree, however, on the major strategies and correctives to be sought. The health care system is a feeding trough for many powerful interests who will not give up their sources of revenue easily. Reform usually comes most smoothly when there are large expansions in investment and most involved parties see themselves gaining through change. Health reforms in the context of budgetary stringency and a large federal deficit can't be lubricated by large giveaways. Economic constraints will make it difficult to achieve the necessary consensus for the changes needed.

Reforming our health insurance system is only one aspect of the health care challenge. While financing provides the framework for care, the values and goals for the health enterprise remain undefined. Financial reform is a necessary enabling condition, but it is essential to be clear on the functions, roles, and goals of our institutions, programs, and professionals. In this book, I argue that we require nothing less than a transformation of the medical paradigm and in the ways that we address health affairs. I believe that we must increasingly turn our attention to devising strategies at both the community and individual levels for preventing illness and maximizing function so that individuals who are sick can continue their preferred activities with as little disruption and discomfort as possible. An increasing component of medical work deals with chronic disease and disabilities, but we have yet to develop a longitudinal approach to clinical care that is sufficiently sensitive to the course of disease in its psychosocial and community context.

This collection of ten essays, organized into four sections, is based largely on previously published work. The essays, some integrated with one another and presented in revised form, appeared in about a dozen different publications representing such diverse disciplines as medical care, sociology, law, political science, health policy, pediatrics, and psychiatry. By bringing them together, I not only make them readily accessible to the social science and health audience but also present them in a way that offers a broader and more forceful statement than the individual essays or subsets of them do.

In Part I, I show how technology, forms of organization and reimbursement, and population expectations have led us into our current fix. I examine how efforts to maintain a highly pluralistic privatized system resulted in a pattern of regulated micromanagement that amazes even those doctors and other health professionals working in highly bureaucratized health systems in other countries.

In arguing for a new approach, I maintain that costs will never be brought under control without a budgetary ceiling. Although I favor a Canadian-like plan, I find such an approach unlikely in the United States context, as I explain in the first essay, and so I discuss other reform alternatives as well. The second essay examines the changing role of physicians and considers the argument that physicians are increasingly proletarianized, a contention commonly made. I argue that while physician autonomy is being eroded in certain areas, medicine as a cultural paradigm is more powerful than ever and that medical perspectives continue to dominate many aspects of American life. In the third essay, I pick up on an earlier theme to consider how to constrain costs in a manner sensitive to clinical issues and patient needs. I argue that implicit rationing—that is, establishing budgetary limits within which health professionals must work—offers the most realistic, appropriate and nonintrusive way to allocate services. Because patient populations are heterogeneous, and many medical interventions are uncertain, the clinical decision-making process is iterative. An effective and sensible health care rationing scheme must take into account the need for flexible response. I suggest that future rationing must involve a blend of approaches, and the real debate should focus on how to best achieve a proper mix.

The second set of essays begins to define what I mean by a new health paradigm. I examine current research that shows that health is truly a social phenomenon and very much influenced by individuals' sense of social well-being. I explore the need for a broader strategy to promote health and prevent illness and one that views the challenge of health in terms of functional capacity and quality of life. I examine the robust relationship between socioeconomic status and health and some of the intervening variables that may help explain why individuals with relatively little education and income fare poorly on most indicators of health, disease, and mortality.

In Part III, I turn to a consideration of three special populations: adolescents, persons with mental illness, and the elderly. Each of these populations exemplify the failures of our current medical care paradigm and the need for a new approach. The challenge in adolescence is the "new morbidity." Adolescents have little serious physical illness but are at risk for substance abuse, violence, early pregnancy, sexually transmitted diseases, and other patterns that arise from their social milieu, family disorganization, peer group pressures, and community breakdown. I examine various community initiatives that may be helpful in reducing risk and building competence. The chapter on the mentally ill, written with David Rochefort of Northeastern University, explores how we created the mess we currently face in the care of persons with serious and persistent mental illness. We demonstrate that much of the confusion and neglect that characterizes this population flows from our way of dealing with health and welfare issues, which makes services fragmentation inevitable. We suggest that if integration of services is a goal, as it should be, much stronger and coordinated initiatives are needed than those that usually prevail. Similar patterns are addressed in the care for the sick elderly, particularly in relationship to the need for a coherent long-term care approach.

The final section seeks to relate various themes discussed in the book to the unfolding efforts to reform our health insurance system. Given the complexity of our health care system and the diversity of groups involved, it is difficult to develop a dialogue that allows the debate to constructively advance. The debate reflects a very simplified version of reality and tends to focus on generic issues of interest to the largest number of participants. But in addressing the most common generic issues affecting the generally healthy populations, it is relatively easy to overlook the special needs and difficulties of smaller but especially vulnerable populations. It is also easy to ignore potential initiatives that don't readily fall within the traditional health paradigm. The dilemma is that the debate must be of interest to sufficient numbers of people to build the needed momentum for change, but the proposed solutions for the majority of the population may not speak to the special needs of persons with physical disabilities, mental illness, developmental disabilities, and the like. As the inevitable political compromises take place in efforts to achieve a reasonable consensus, great care must be taken to insure that the needs of smaller, less visible, and less powerful groups are thoughtfully addressed as well. The irony is that in the process of making the system of care better for most, some inevitably come out worse off. Vigilance for especially vulnerable groups must be a high priority.

The book also includes an appendix with two papers that focus on issues in the social sciences of medicine and its contrasting cultures. These essays don't neatly fit the main part of the book. The appendix looks inwardly at the disciplines that do much of the research on health and health care and may be of more interest to social scientists who work in medicine than to the broader public. While these are not technical papers and could be read profitably by the general reader, they are not central to the main thesis of this book. I include them because the social science disciplines discussed contribute importantly to framing issues and the terms of public debate over health, and influence the climate of opinion among the educated public.

It is clear enough that concerns about costs, and the associated ascendancy of economics and finance in discussions of health care, have significantly narrowed how we frame health care issues and the context of the health care debate. Yet, as we look to the future, it is inevitable that the debate will be broadened again. Financing structures are essential conditions for enabling the processes of care, but within any framework there are innumerable questions of values and objectives and how they intersect with issues of class, race, gender, and ethnicity. Nor can we ignore the relations between the structures we develop and the arrangements of power, influence, and control in our society. In the appendix, I suggest that if we did not have a rich social science of medicine we would have to invent one because the health system is in some sense a mirror to the values, tensions, and conflicts that characterize our daily lives. Such influences play a major role in the morbidity the system encounters and the shape of health care services. Greater awareness of the issues can help us define more effective and more humane policies.

PART I

The Medical Care System in Disarray

1

The American Medical Care System

My purpose here is to examine some future possible structures for
health care. To do this responsibly requires consideration of how the
health care system can play an increased role in maintaining and enhancing health and function and not simply focus on treating disease. In
recognizing the health-producing potential of the health system, we must
nevertheless keep in mind that macroforces set limits on the contributions
of health services. Medical care cannot compensate for economic
deprivation, social disorganization, personal alienation, and low levels
of education and social integration, although it can offer assistance and
support for those affected. These situations of deprivation impoverish
human lives, incite conflict and violence, contribute to deleterious personal and group behavior, and explain many of the observable disparities
in health status. Achieving more equal health outcomes requires a more
equitable society in which all groups have a stake.

The theme of this chapter is that while American medicine has in the
past several decades undergone extraordinary changes in technology,
economic growth, organizational arrangements, and government involvement, its core culture has remained relatively stable and resilient.
Despite all the changes, the system maintains an individual as compared
with a community perspective, an emphasis on aggressive intervention,
and a focus on cures and more narrow biomedical concerns. Despite
many intrusions from government and other third parties, medicine, and
particularly its technical subspecialties, retain their dominance although
one might have expected the growth of countervailing influences to have

Adapted from "The American Health Care System and Its Future," *Medical Care Review* 50, no. 1
(Spring 1993) with permission of the J.B. Lippincott Co.

modified the power base and directions of medical work more substantially (see chap. 2).

We need an alternative view of medicine, one organized around a framework of equitable access in relation to need, greater sensitivity to the needs of the disadvantaged, a process of care that seeks to promote and support function among the chronically ill and disabled, and a greater focus on prevention and community health. This does not imply denigration of the extraordinary developments that advances in science and technology have made possible. It requires, however, that these be applied within a broader framework of values and priorities. None of these caring goals are foreign to medicine, and each are pursued now somewhere in our large and heterogeneous system of care. The challenge is to elevate the priority of elements that are now tangential to the main course of health care activity.

As we look to the future it is also clear that much about medicine will inevitably change—patterns of disease, the scope of our knowledge, technologies, economic organization, patient expectations, and much more. Unexpected problems and new diseases will emerge, for as René Dubos (1959) reminded us, "fitness requires never-ending efforts of adaptation to the total environment, which is ever changing." The emergence of other new diseases, such as AIDS, with their devastating consequences for individuals and societies, will pose unexpected challenges. The future is unpredictable, and I am deeply skeptical of efforts to foresee it. It depends not only on changes in the natural environment and emerging strains of viruses and bacteria but also on the emergence of new social and environmental problems and related morbidity. It also depends on the evolution of our economy and politics, and how we manage new developments in science and technology.

Effectiveness depends both on the content of what health professionals do and the financial and organizational frameworks within which their work is embedded. Although I present a view of what is needed, I see myself as a "despairing optimist," a designation René Dubos adopted some years ago. On the one hand, only a fool fails to recognize the interests with a stake in current perspectives and foci, and their determination to resist fundamental change, a cause for despair. On the other hand, our rich professional and material resources and the large numbers of dedicated, creative, and energetic health professionals committed to change offer hope for a more constructive future.

The Culture of American Medical Care:
Technology and Interventionism

Technology is a process of organizing inputs to achieve specified outcomes, but to most people technology is synonymous with hardware—the artificial kidney, electronic monitoring, computerized tomography (CT), nuclear magnetic resonance (NMR), and lithotripters. This common confusion is symptomatic of the difficulties we face in mobilizing the vast resources we expend on health care toward the design of an effective, affordable, and equitable framework of care for all Americans.

We well know, and no one seriously contests the fact, that the prevalent incentives—whether measured by remuneration, influence, or public respect—reward those who engage their energies in the development and application of new hardware. We understand that physician payment rewards technical and invasive procedures far more handsomely than it rewards thoughtful decision making, sensitive communication, and efforts to educate and promote health. Recent work on a resource-based relative-value scale for physician payment by Hsiao and his colleagues (1988) indicated that one of the most undervalued services was an initial office visit by a healthy adult to an internist. In this extreme case, the mean Medicare charge relative to the resource-based relative value was 18 percent. The comparable figures for insertion of a pacemaker or for repair on an inguinal hernia were 232 percent and 154 percent. As Hsiao and his associates noted, "invasive procedures are typically compensated at more than double the rate of evaluation and management services, when both consume the same resource inputs" (p. 881). We also see that neonatal hardware captures the imagination of both professionals and the public far more than the seemingly routine and mundane efforts to oversee healthy development, monitor risks among pregnant women, or ensure that children are properly immunized. And we know that efforts to implant devices in the elderly or image the brain of schizophrenics seem far more exciting than organizing the complex social resources and financing arrangements essential to long-term community care that sustain function and quality of life for the elderly, the seriously mentally ill, and other populations.

Noting these tendencies (some would say aberrations) in no way diminishes the extraordinary advances made thus far in biomedical sciences and technology or those advances yet to come. Nor do I seek to minimize the enormous value and comfort some new technical advances represent (e.g., hip replacements that allow new mobility, implantation of intraocular lenses that facilitate sight, NMR imaging that substitutes for invasive and more dangerous interventions) or the exciting innovations on the horizon. The extraordinary success of so much new hardware, and the potential of new techniques and drugs, excites the imagination of the public as well as the enthusiasm of scientists and health professionals. Surveys of the public persistently show strong support for continued investment in medical technology, and the unequivocal evidence of its successes sets the context for confusion in our values and distortions in our priorities. In large part because of this record of success, tolerance for the use of new hardware is extraordinarily wide, even in the absence of effectiveness or in the presence of more compelling and competing priorities.

Viewed in terms of scientific standards of effectiveness, much of medical care and the sophisticated medical technology on the cutting edge—while valuable under limited circumstances—is used inappropriately. A recent study by RAND investigators on the appropriateness of use of coronary angiography, carotid endarterectomy, and upper gastrointestinal tract endoscopy, using liberal criteria, found that between 17 percent and 32 percent of use was inappropriate (Chassin et al. 1987). Many other technologies and interventions have been criticized as useless or worse. Consider, for example, the widespread adoption in the 1970s of intrapartum electronic fetal heart rate monitoring, believed to detect fetal hypoxia in a timely manner, thus preventing death and neurological damage. Numerous randomized controlled trials have failed to show any benefit relative to the traditional method of auscultation, but fetal monitoring is now almost universal (Shy, Larson et al. 1987). Defenders of the technology have believed that its value is more evident with premature infants, but a randomized controlled trial and follow-up study have failed to confirm this. Instead, fetal monitoring has been associated with increased cesarean sections and forceps deliveries. Shy and his colleagues (Shy, Luthy et al. 1990) found "an unanticipated 2.9-fold increase in the odds of having cerebral palsy among infants weighing 1,750g or less who had electronic fetal monitoring as compared to infants who had periodic auscultation. This increase was observed at each of the three study hospitals" (p. 592). The cerebral palsy finding may be an artifact, but it seems more clear that fetal monitoring may result in exaggerated assessments of fetal distress and may stimulate unnecessary and risky medical interventions.

Typically, young physicians and nurses are no longer taught traditional auscultation, leading to total dependence on instruments for electronic monitoring, and new practitioners have little experience in acquiring basic clinical skills, a particular problem for those from developing nations trained in the United States. Similarly, the claims for electrocardiographic monitoring and the expensive development of intensive coronary care have not been supported by several randomized clinical trials (Waitzkin 1979). The circumstances surrounding electronic monitoring of internal organs apply as well to many other commonly used technologies.

A wide range of factors sustain an emphasis on technical procedures even when the procedures are uncertain and ineffective, accounting in part for the enormous variations across practice areas. Clinicians are more guided by their experiences than by abstract studies and often feel confident on the basis of particular instances when the procedures used have been helpful. Our systems of payment typically make it economically rewarding to use sophisticated equipment and procedures in instances of uncertainty. Further, increasing awareness stimulated by mass media coverage of new procedures and hardware commonly brings patients to medical settings convinced of the value of new technical approaches. The failure to use such technologies, even when unwarranted by the scientific literature, may put physicians and hospitals at risk of malpractice litigation. Moreover, once these technologies are introduced, there is strong incentive for maintaining their use—for both the medical manufacturers and the professionals who use the products. Thus, we have woven a pattern of interests and incentives that makes it difficult to forgo technical hardware and procedures in instances of uncertainty.

Some years ago, Victor Fuchs (1968) described the bias among physicians toward the technological imperative, the tendency to try everything possible on behalf of the patient that offered any potential, however small. In the subsequent years there has been much discussion of managing care and related concepts such as cost-effectiveness, balancing, and rationing. Capitated systems such as HMOs have had clear incentives to moderate use of expensive modalities, in contrast to fee-for-service medicine where there is more encouragement to be technically aggressive in marginal situations (Luft 1987). The introduction of new technologies continues unabated, however, encouraged by aggressive marketing by industries that manufacture and sell medical and hospital equipment and drugs (Waitzkin 1983), by economic incentives, and by public and professional support.

The aggressiveness of American medicine in the uses of technology transcends skillful marketing or even the economic incentives that make its adoption highly profitable. American culture is individualistic and intervention-oriented, and we act as if technology offers potential solutions to almost any of our problems (Payer 1988). New technology diffuses rapidly, often well before there is any systematic evidence of its value, and almost always before its cost-effectiveness is assessed.

Culture is, of course, difficult to change, particularly when it is reinforced by occasional spectacular successes, aggressive marketing, and profitable opportunities. In the past twenty-five years, American hospitals grew enormously, capitalizing on the opportunities of federal funding, first through the Hill-Burton Program and then through favorable incentives for writing off depreciation under the Medicare program. Instead of paying for depreciation in terms of original cost, depreciation was defined in terms of current replacement costs, giving hospitals considerable incentive for further expansion. In addition, 2 percent of reimbursable costs was added under Medicare for what was viewed as necessary capital enhancement and for-profit hospitals were additionally guaranteed a substantial return on equity capital as an allowable cost (Stevens 1989:296–97). These opportunities stimulated enormous capital expansion by allowing hospitals to pass the costs on to government and other third party payers. Stimulated by a competitive, entrepreneurial ethos, the hospital sector grew in a fashion that offered state-of-the-art technology almost everywhere, with large duplication of expensive technologies and specialized units that were frequently underutilized. Many of these little used facilities, however, could not provide care of comparative quality to those carrying out a higher volume of specialized procedures. The incentive structure that affects adoption and use of new technology encourages utilization where little benefit is expected. This is true of both ordinary diagnostic tests that are often used as well as "big ticket" items such as imaging studies and expensive surgical interventions.

Much of the success of American medicine derives from its openness to new cutting-edge technologies, and its aggressive pursuit through research and development of innovative medical, surgical, and drug treatments. The causes of most major diseases remain unknown, and many of our interventions are what Lewis Thomas has called "half-way" technologies (Thomas 1977). Many have faith that with increased basic scientific knowledge our technological approaches will become more specific and targeted, and as a result more cost-effective, and that fully curative technologies will substitute for less efficient halfway approaches. Moreover, with increased technological capacities, it seems reasonable to anticipate that many commonly used technologies will become less expensive over time.

Warner (1987) has suggested that an appropriate set of economic incentives could lead to substantial development of cost-saving approaches and increased motivation among health professionals to seek less costly alternatives. There is not much indication of any strong tendency in this direction, although the Health Care Financing Agency has recently announced its intention to consider cost-effectiveness of new technologies in its reimbursement decisions. In theory, technical advances, such as in the development of computers that made access to sophisticated information bases relatively inexpensive, should induce efficiency and cost savings. But translating an increased capacity for efficiency into cost savings is a managerial and organizational process, and the introduction of computerization in business did not result in the anticipated reductions in secretarial and clerical personnel. Achieving efficiency requires a change in attitudes, a major barrier to changing the behavior. Economic incentives can help change the behavior of physicians (Eisenberg 1991), but not as much or as quickly as many people assume.

There are those who believe that the chances of modifying priorities are much better at the level at which research and development (R&D) investment is targeted than at the point at which therapies become clinically applicable. They argue that we should not invest in researching new technologies that primarily extend old age and debility because such technologies are likely to have social costs that exceed benefits. And, certainly, it can be argued compellingly that a larger proportion of our vast R&D investments should go to such issues as prevention and behavior and health. Life-styles and social risk factors affect health, longevity, and function far more than those on which the biomedical establishment focuses.

However plausible this position may appear, it has two basic practical weaknesses. First, it is unlikely that our politics will allow it—as evidenced recently by Congress's intimidation of the National Institutes of Health when the NIH decided to phase out its research program on the artificial heart. It is difficult to imagine the American public accepting any policy that reduces our efforts to deal with such diseases of old age as Alzheimers, stroke, cardiovascular disease, and the like. A more serious limitation of this argument is its neglect of the way scientific development proceeds and the dynamics of discovery. Science develops momentum around innovative and exciting ideas and technical developments that allow new options to be pursued, not on the basis of judgments that define what would be the most cost-effective or of the greatest social value. Much of the product of science is serendipitous and not easily programmed. We have, of course, waged all-out war on problems such as cancer, but the notable failures of such shotgun approaches in contrast to more orderly scientific development would suggest that we might have considerable difficulty programming future scientific advances to our specifications.

Looking to the future, I doubt that new technologies will solve our most pressing dilemmas. I have no doubt that there will be new cures and major advances in noninvasive diagnostics, in the development of synthetic body parts, in miniaturization, in computerization, and in the collection and processing of medical information. I anticipate new vaccines, drugs, prosthetics, and materials. Computerization at the bedside will make note-writing and medical records obsolete, and information retrieval will be rapid and efficient. I am confident that these changes will contribute to improved care if used wisely, but anticipate that aggregate costs will increase as well. I am sure that we will have fundamental breakthroughs in some areas, and that some new technologies will be cost-saving. Overall, however, I anticipate many more expensive halfway measures that add small increments to health at large cost. Many chronic conditions, such as cardiovascular disease, develop over a lifetime, and it is naive to expect a future "quick fix."

The danger is that the excitement of new technologies will divert us from the more simple organizational measures that promote prevention and that reach out to underserved people, provide ready access to basic health monitoring, health education, primary medical care, and appropriate referral. We have much new to learn but we also have to learn better to implement what we already know.

Goals for a Health Care System

Much of the progress in medicine in this century came from pursuing a relatively narrow paradigm—the concept of specific etiology—which was a powerful model for identifying causes of infectious disease that could be controlled (Mechanic 1978a). As the disease picture changes, and as the population ages, the major causes of disease and disability are long-term chronic conditions resulting from many causes and not susceptible to a "magic bullet." We need a health care system that is responsive to the need for prevention and continuing care for the chronically ill that maintains and enhances the ability to function.

Changing Societal Structures

Medical care has a broad role in modern societies, in part a result of the erosion of the influence of religion, the family, and other major institutions. At present rates, two-fifths of U.S. children will experience family breakups before age eighteen (Cherlin et al. 1991), and more adults than ever before live in single-person households with few social supports. Religion is a less powerful influence on people's lives, and problems that in the past would have been appropriate for the family or the church to deal with require human services interventions, including medical care. The boundaries of medicine have expanded enormously in recent decades, increasingly dealing with a wide range of social and psychosocial problems traditionally handled in other ways. Physicians deal with many patients whose visits are motivated by feelings of depression, anxiety, worry, and social isolation. Depression and other adverse psychological states increase perceptions of ill health, disability, and utilization of health care services. Recent findings from the Medical Outcomes Study, a large multisite investigation of more than 11,000 outpatients, indicate that depression is more disabling than many of the most serious chronic medical conditions that physicians typically deal with (Wells et al. 1989), thus requiring attention in the primary health care sector. In addition, growing evidence of the extent to which personal behavior and life-styles relate to risks of morbidity and death (Assistant

Secretary for Health 1979, 1990) suggests that physicians must take broader responsibility for patient education and efforts to modify behavior.

The Role of Prevention

Despite much lip service to prevention, we have done relatively little to educate physicians to appropriately use behavior modification to reduce noxious behaviors, or to enable them in their practices to devote the time necessary for serious health maintenance. Much of prevention, of course, requires broad educational efforts at the community level and the encouragement of everyday family, work, and recreational activities in a manner promotive of positive health outcomes. Successful prevention is a product of culture and the social arrangements of everyday activities (Mechanic 1990). But physicians commonly encounter patients when they are anxious and worried, and when they are particularly amenable to influence (Frank and Frank 1991). The physician still remains a respected and credible authority figure who can have an important influence on behaviors such as smoking, diet, and substance abuse. The quality of doctor-patient interaction is also important in achieving satisfactory understanding and adherence to medical advice more generally. Existing studies suggest that successful behavior modification requires appropriate knowledge, coping skills to overcome barriers to the enactment of the desired behavior, and continuing reinforcement for the emergent behavior changes (Mechanic 1991a; Mechanic and Aiken 1991; Leventhal et al. 1985). A variety of techniques are available to assist physicians in achieving successful adherence to prescribed medical regimens (Svarstad 1986).

A key element in many of the educational and preventive approaches is sufficient time to communicate clearly, to elicit questions, and to provide appropriate feedback. But in medicine, time is money, and educational efforts are not remunerative. Although ultimate conversion to a resource-based relative-value system may eventually give higher value to cognitive and educational services, the prospects of making such services competitive with more technical interventions are not promising. Nor is capitated care a particularly likely solution, since physicians in HMOs work under strict time constraints and with cost containment efforts these pressures are likely to increase as well. Preventive educational efforts even within these time constraints may be cost-effective but physicians facing workload pressures may not see the issue in this light.

Physicians also often experience a sense of futility in helping patients cope with problems and disadvantages that medicine can do little about, and they commonly deflect discussion away from such issues (Waitzkin and Britt 1989). Nor do they feel particularly adept at changing complex behavior patterns related to health that are not simply subject to cognitive knowledge or exhortation. In their frustration they often focus on what they know, searching for something they can treat, although the problem they identify or the treatment may not add greatly to the patient's quality of life and may not even be particularly responsive to the patient's complaints. This is seen commonly in the elderly with chronic disease who have many signs of frailty and dysfunction. Too often physicians focus on improving minor identifiable physical problems, readily within their repertoires, rather than on a course of action that might better serve their patients.

Preventive education is one area in which a clinical in contrast to an epidemiological perspective is deceptively discouraging. A very brief counseling session with a physician can decrease the rate of patient smoking. Five percent of patients given counseling for one or two minutes during a routine consultation, reinforced by a four-page pamphlet on how to give up smoking, stopped smoking within one month following the intervention and were abstinent over a one year period (Russell, Wilson et al. 1979). Rates of success can probably be increased further by linking patients to smoking clinics and using nicotine chewing gum (Russell, Stapleton et al. 1987). Even modest change is important because of the noxious effects of long-term cigarette use. Assuming a physician counseled 100 patients, 3 would terminate smoking as a matter of course, and 5 would quit as a result of physician intervention. A 5 percent termination rate relative to the modest aggregate time expended is perhaps one of the most cost-effective things a physician can do, but physician perception will be unduly influenced by the vast majority of patients who do not change their behavior. On the basis of these experienced failures, physicians commonly develop negative attitudes toward health counseling. This, of course, is an excellent reason to insure that young physicians become familiar with the principles of clinical epidemiology.

In future years preventive and educational efforts will require both the increased use of nonphysicians and more creative use of communication technologies. Nurse practitioners do well in primary care in part because they take more time with patients and provide a climate in which patients can comfortably ask questions and provide appropriate feedback. These are important conditions for the successful use of behavioral interventions, and use of physician extenders compensates for most physicians who fail to take the necessary time. Moreover, there is substantial room for creativity in using video and other communication technologies to prepare patients for medical procedures, and to inform them about health issues, their particular illness problems, and ways of living with and managing chronic symptoms. Follow-up to elicit feedback and answer questions is essential for individualized treatment, but good software can reduce the educational demands considerably. Patients spend much unproductive time in hospitals and clinics that could be used constructively for both specific instruction and general health education.

Improved training is certainly important at the level of the individual practitioner, but systems of care must also develop structural alternatives to the imperatives of technical intervention. Some HMOs have developed such alternatives to some degree, including health education, smoking cessation assistance, social support groups, and the like. These additional services are popular among some enrollees and at the margins may help explain why HMOs are chosen in multiple choice situations (Mechanic, Ettel, and Davis 1990). However, such supplemental services, which may be highly cost-effective in capitated programs, may face major obstacles in fee-for-service practice. If they truly are alternatives to some physician care, physicians have disincentives to encourage them. And if, on the other hand, patients may be charged substantially for these additional services, there is a clear disincentive to use them. The concept of trade-off and alternatives, whatever the problem being addressed, is unlikely to work well in systems that pay for care on a piecemeal basis.

A major implication is that payment systems must evolve in close relationship with goals. The beauty of capitation or global budgets is that they provide incentives for cost-saving innovations and eliminate barriers to substituting nonmedical for medical services. Unfortunately, capitation or global budgets in the absence of other incentives and measures for quality assurance can result in mediocre services and poor responsiveness (Mechanic 1974; Glaser 1970; Luft 1987). The evidence argues for a mixed system of reimbursement that builds on the basic advantages of capitation but then uses a complex set of incentives to enhance productivity and responsiveness within the capitation framework. For example, half of the physician's income might come from a core salary or capitation, while the second half could reflect an aggregate of productivity measures, assessment by peers, and periodic sampling of patient satisfaction. Although most of these methods have been used in one context or another, their use in combination has not been well studied.

It is essential that the basis for reimbursement be multifaceted and complex so that it is not easily manipulated by providers seeking to maximize their remuneration. Simply rewarding productivity or patient satisfaction or peer esteem encourages manipulation. Combining the criteria makes it difficult to "game" the system and has the advantage of rewarding varied bases of performance, each of which is important.

The Need for Long-term Care

Chronic disease is concentrated in later life and much of medical care focuses on treatment of the elderly, where the challenge is typically less one of effecting cures and more of enhancing function. Since the end of the Second World War U.S. medical care has turned its major attention to chronic disease (Fox 1986), but care continues to be focused more on acute episodes and exacerbations of disease than on the longitudinal issues necessary to maximize function. Between 1960 and 1980, persons in the age group over eighty-five increased 174 percent, and a 110 percent increase is expected between 1980 and the end of the century (Rice and Feldman 1983). By the year 2000, more than one-quarter of the expected elderly population of 36 million will be older than age eighty. As we look further into the future, when the baby boom birth cohorts begin to approach old age, beginning in about twenty years, the elderly population is expected to constitute 17 percent of the population (Office of Technology Assessment 1985). As the numbers of old-old patients increase, the importance of strategies that allow individuals to retain independence becomes even more apparent.

The changing demography of the population poses a significant need for a national long-term care policy. In the absence of such a policy Medicaid has been the de facto federal long-term care program with 14 percent of elderly Medicaid beneficiaries accounting for 36 percent of

Medicaid payments, two-thirds of which go for nursing home care (Ball and Bethell 1989). Many elderly who enter nursing homes rapidly deplete their resources and become eligible for Medicaid, drawing resources away from other important Medicaid populations. The share of nursing home care financed by the federal government actually decreased from 53.4 percent in 1981 to 48.6 percent in 1988 (Office of National Cost Estimates 1990). Most nursing home care continues to be financed privately, typically from personal and family resources rather than insurance. The magnitude of expenditures for services provided by non-facility-based home care agencies has increased rapidly from $1.3 billion in 1980 to $4.4 billion in 1988 (Office of National Cost Estimates 1990). These estimates, however, exclude expanded services such as adult day care, respite care, and supportive social services. Rivlin and Wiener (1988) estimated annual spending under an expanded definition of home care services as $8.7 billion. Needs for such services, and related financing, are likely to grow dramatically in coming decades.

There has been some development of private long-term care insurance in recent years but such insurance is costly, has significant eligibility restrictions, has limited coverage, provides inadequate and limited duration of benefits, and involves uncertainties concerning renewability (Ball and Bethell 1989). Although long-term insurance may contribute toward part of an ultimate solution, it is not a viable strategy by itself (Rivlin and Wiener 1988; Ball and Bethell 1989). Alternatively, budgetary constraints and uncertainties of predicting cost have made government reluctant to assume responsibility. The Pepper Commission (1990) recommended a long-term care program including a requirement for insurance for home and community-based care and for the first three months of nursing home care, and a floor to protect persons with long nursing stays against impoverishment. The federal government, under this proposal, would subsidize persons with low incomes. The Commission estimated that the program would cover 4.4 million people at an increased federal cost of $42.8 billion. Others have suggested developing a long-term care program under Medicare, for example a part C (Somers 1987) or expanding Medicaid eligibility (Pauly 1988).

There is little consensus on the philosophy of a long-term care policy and the emphasis to be given to providing front-end care versus protecting private assets through catastrophic insurance. A reasonable federal role is to insure that persons receive needed care, while the protection of personal assets may be more properly a role for the private sector. Most agree, however, that a financially viable long-term care program would require considerable sharing of government and private responsibility, cost-sharing in relationship to capacity to pay, and stringent gatekeeping to insure financial viability of the program. Effective gatekeeping is particularly important as the service mix comes to include more home and community care because it is in these areas that substitution of formal services for informal care is most likely to occur. Effective long-term care policy will require the capacity to target for services groups that would have a high risk of institutionalization without intervention (Weissert 1991). It is well-known that the extension of new community services attracts new clients who are not of highest risk for institutional care but such services mostly supplement informal services rather than substitute for them (Kemper et al. 1987; Tennstedt and McKinlay 1989). Ball and Bethell (1989) have suggested a framework of goals for long-term care: a universal plan integrated into our Social Security system, into which most contribute; coverage of anyone who becomes chronically ill or disabled; coverage of both home and nursing home care; service to both patients and informal caregivers; emphasis on support for independent functioning; direct payment for necessary services; encouragement of alternative long-term care services; cost-sharing; and stringent cost and quality controls. It seems evident that development of a long-term care policy will continue its long gestation.

Significant future efforts in medicine will be focused on disabilities and their secondary complications due both to the aging of the population and the increasing demands of persons with disabilities that their concerns be given greater centrality in medical care processes. It is difficult to reach a firm estimate of the prevalence of disabilities because of a multiplicity of definitions. The National Health Interview Survey, based on a sampling of the noninstitutionalized population, reported that in 1988 more than 33 million people (13.7 percent of the noninstitutionalized population) had an activity limitation resulting from chronic conditions (Institute of Medicine 1991). Almost 10 million of these people cannot carry out the major activity for someone of their age, and more than another 13 million are limited in the amount or kind of major activities they can carry out. Such limitations increase with age, affecting almost two-fifths of the population seventy years or older.

Integration of Medicine and Public Health

Many of the influences associated with disability and death derive from social conditions and personal risk factors that are potentially preventable to a significant degree through social policy interventions and behavioral modifications. Accidents, suicide, and homicide account for increasing proportions of deaths, particularly among young people, and much of premature morbidity and mortality is linked to abuse of alcohol and drugs, smoking, poor nutrition, and high-risk behavior associated with HIV infection. It is difficult to anticipate how our society will deal in the future with such conflict-laden issues as jobs, the distribution of income, toxic waste and environmental issues, abortion, tobacco, gun control, and numerous other factors related to health outcomes. It is more predictable that major efforts will be launched to modify personal risk factors. Creating a tobacco-free society by itself would have enormous implications for the magnitude of disease, disability, and death and for the demand for specific types of specialized medical care (Warner 1987). Whatever the political likelihood of banning tobacco or lack thereof, progress will continue in changing the culture surrounding smoking and the prevalence of smoking in the population, and the conditions affecting the prevalence of other health damaging behaviors as well.

These changes, and their influences on patterns of disease occurrence will modify the clinical picture seen by the average physician. At one end of the age spectrum, the challenge will be the "new morbidities," associated with personal and social disruptions and alienation, and family dissolution. Much illness, however, will be delayed to later life where the crucial challenge will be to maintain function in numerous ways, such as by controlling urinary incontinence, teaching coping techniques for dealing with decrements in memory and orientation, and aiding social attachments for persons whose personal networks have been depleted. Traditional medical approaches are ill-suited to such impending health challenges and these tasks will require major modifications in professional education and the design of medical practice (Robert Wood Johnson Foundation 1991).

The concerns of public health and medicine need better integration in the years ahead. If medicine is to be an effective instrument for maintaining and enhancing health, substantial attention to populations and the potentialities for prevention are required. Relatively few resources in either research or practice go to broad community preventive programs or even to individual patient interventions, in contrast to very intensive remedial medical care. Medicine is in essence an individual treatment endeavor and will remain so. But it is foolish and futile to spend increasingly vast resources to save damaged lives, while giving little attention to the conditions that erode reasonable life chances and healthful function.

The pessimism many physicians feel about prevention undermines efforts in areas in which valuable strategies and technologies are available, as in the smoking counseling example. Also, data from the U.S. immunization survey indicate that approximately two-fifths of children one to four years of age are not immunized against measles, rubella, polio, or mumps.* DPT nonimmunization reported rates are somewhat lower, 35 percent, but still unacceptable. Among nonwhites, a group at greater risk because of poverty and less adequate nutrition, less than half reported being immunized for any of the above diseases (National Center for Health Statistics 1991). The recent outbreak of measles in a number of major cities, and the occurrence of preventable deaths, attests to our neglect. The incongruency between current efforts to save low birth weight children and the limited efforts to deliver inexpensive and routine preventive measures to high-risk mothers and children raises grave questions about our priorities and wisdom. Neonatal intensive care for an infant weighing 1500 grams costs on average $26,000 (Office of Technology Assessment 1987), and such low birthweight infants predominate in high-risk disadvantaged groups. Concentrated efforts to identify high-risk mothers and provide appropriate prenatal and child care is probably in the long run far more effective than high-technology care concentrated on one early stage of infant development.

Prevention, of course, is not a simple matter, nor is it always cost-effective. In many instances we lack the knowledge and technology to successfully modify disease risk or change behavior. In other areas, the risks are of such low probability, and the target populations so large, that even preventive efforts that are inexpensive per individual administration

---

* These data are reported in the household interview survey, and probably underestimate actual vaccination. Data from 1985, with a subsample that consulted vaccination records, show higher rates, more in the vicinity of 75 percent for most vaccinations, and 87 percent for DPT. Among nonwhites, rates vary from three-fifths to two-thirds, with the exception of DPT where 75 percent report vaccinations (National Center for Health Statistics 1991:table 42).

are extraordinarily costly in the aggregate relative to the gains achieved and do not give value for the money (Russell 1986). Yet the future of medicine, and the value of the enormous resources we expend, depend on the success of the strategies we develop to prevent disease, limit disability, enhance function, support and maintain the chronically ill and disabled, and contribute to a better quality of life.

The Challenge of Disadvantage

Sophisticated observers from other nations admire the scientific and technological accomplishments of American medicine but are incredulous that we can expend such vast resources and still have large segments of our population uninsured and underinsured and persistent barriers to offering every person access to basic health care. It seems peculiar, indeed, that a nation that spends so much on health care tolerates the massive inequalities in care that characterize the American situation.

In an extraordinary illustration of the consequences of inequality, McCord and Freeman (1990) examined mortality rates in the central Harlem health district in New York City for the period 1979 to 1981. This community is 96 percent black and two-fifths of the population live below the poverty line. Mortality in central Harlem was more than double that of the American population, and survival to age sixty-five for black men was lower than in Bangladesh, an exceedingly poor, undeveloped country. Excess deaths in Harlem relative to the American population were primarily explained by cardiovascular disease, cirrhosis, homicide, and neoplasms. Deaths due to drug dependency, homicide, alcohol use, and cirrhosis were from 10 to 283 times more likely to occur in Harlem than in the national population. Although the Harlem health district had the highest mortality in the city, 54 of the 353 health districts in the city had at least double the expected deaths using the American population as a standard. All but one of these health districts were largely black and Hispanic impoverished areas. These findings reaffirm the observations of the Task Force of the Secretary of the Department of Health and Human Services (*Report of the Secretary's Task Force Task Force on Black and Minority Health 1985*) who estimated 42.5 percent excess deaths among the black population in the United States in the period 1979–81, and there is little evidence of improvement since then. While limited access to medical care plays some role in explaining health disadvantage, it is clear that much of the observed morbidity, disability, and mortality is due substantially to the social and economic circumstances of blacks, other minorities, and the disadvantaged more generally (Bunker, Gomby, et al. 1989).

Persons with lower socioeconomic status are at higher risk of morbidity, disability and mortality than those more affluent (Bunker, Gomby and Kehrer 1989; Dutton 1986). They are exposed to more risk factors, are more vulnerable to them when exposed, and have less resources to counter harmful situations. They have less access to medical care relative to need than the more advantaged, and face many barriers in receiving services routinely available to more affluent patients, such as prenatal and child care and preventive services. The poor, and especially poor black and Hispanic populations in large cities, disproportionately receive care from emergency rooms and hospital outpatient clinics, a pattern that interferes with continuity, preventive appraisals and interventions, and health maintenance. Such episodic care typically involves long waiting times, little follow-up and poor coordination of care. Though much care for the disadvantaged is hospital-based, they are less likely than affluent persons to be referred to specialized care and "cutting edge" treatments for such conditions as cancer, heart disease, and mental disorder (Mechanic and Aiken, 1989). The dynamics of differential referral processes are not fully clear, but a major factor affecting differences in treatment is lack of insurance or public insurance such as Medicaid that pays physicians much less than other insurance programs (Hadley, Steinberg, and Feder 1991).

It has been apparent for decades that the emergency and episodic treatment characterizing so much of the care of disadvantaged groups is extraordinarily wasteful, because continuity in care is important in dealing with their complex sociomedical problems. Conversely, the evidence is quite impressive from studies of community health centers that well-organized basic services can contribute importantly to the health of these populations, reduce morbidity, and increase patient satisfaction (Dutton 1986; Freeman, Kiecolt, and Allen 1982). We continue to lose ground in organizing primary care services for the disadvantaged. In the 1990s, we will have to resurrect the commitment that led to the development of the Office of Economic Opportunity health centers in the 1960s.

A major advantage of the community health approach is that it views medical problems in their larger social context, and thus, the approach is more responsive to living conditions that affect the course of illness, secondary complications, and the ability of patients to adhere to medical advice. Such health programs are more likely to engage in outreach efforts to identify needs and to assist patients in gaining eligibility for other types of assistance they require or even in community development efforts. In poverty areas, the separation between medical care and other types of basic assistance patients need—education, sanitation, food supplies—present major barriers to achieving effective care outcomes. The community approach to care is an old model, but its relevance for disadvantaged populations is as great as ever (Kark and Steuart 1962; Geiger 1984).

In the 1960s the nation was focused on issues of access to health care and other welfare entitlements and in meeting the needs of disadvantaged populations. As the emphasis turned to cost containment in the 1970s, attention to these priorities declined and welfare efforts were eroded or failed to keep pace with the growth of the poor population. The erosion of insurance places particular stress on public hospitals and a segment of nonprofit general hospitals that provide substantial care for indigent persons. Access is again a salient issue on the national and state agendas, but in a more complex context of budget deficits and cost-containment pressures. In the interim, we have lost sight of the extraordinary potential of community health care centers to wage a multifaceted attack on the devastating conditions existing in our urban ghettos.

The Evolution of Current Dilemmas

American health care as we know it is largely a post-World War II phenomenon. In 1940 the United States spent $4 billion on health, 4 percent of GNP. By 1950, as a result of the enormous postwar economic growth and inflation, expenditures tripled but expenditures as a proportion of GNP rose only modestly to 4.5 percent. In the post-1955 years, with the growth of health insurance, total health expenditures accelerated more rapidly than GNP, beginning an upward trajectory that continues (National Center for Health Statistics 1991:184). The introduction of Medicare and Medicaid in 1966, greatly expanding the numbers of people covered by insurance under an open-ended reimbursement system, accelerated the rate of health expenditures, so that by 1989, the latest year for which definitive figures are available, expenditures had risen to

$604 billion, 11.6 percent of GNP, and $2354 per capita (Lazenby and Letsch 1990:table 103). Unofficial estimates put the 1992 figure at about $814 billion.

At various points in American history, there were strong efforts to develop a national system of health coverage. President Truman asked Congress to pass a national health program, based on models that had been germinating throughout the 1930s. Opponents of a national system supported and encouraged private hospital insurance as an alternative, a pattern developing since the Great Depression. Blue Cross and Blue Shield's rapid growth in the 1950s and 1960s helped to deflate momentum for a federally sponsored system. The decision by the War Labor Board in 1942 to allow fringe benefits of up to 5 percent of wages, under a wage controlled situation, encouraged health insurance coverage (Stevens 1989:259). Nonprofit and commercial health insurance could expand rapidly in the post-World War II years because health coverage became an important part of fringe benefit programs associated with employment, and workers could get health benefits in excess of what they could get in increased wages because of tax advantages. Individuals outside the employment system were least protected, the elderly being the most visible and politically important subgroup. In the political debates of the early 1960s over health coverage for the elderly, sagacious political maneuvering by Wilbur Mills, with the assistance of Wilbur Cohen, resulted in the enactment of Medicare and Medicaid in 1965 (Marmor 1973).

In reflecting on the "play-by-play" relating to the enactment of these programs, Wilbur Cohen noted that while he "had been a strong advocate of a comprehensive and universal nationwide health insurance plan since 1940," he accepted the "desirability of learning by doing . . . and of resolving problems arising from the unintended consequences of legislative behavior that affected human and institutional behavior." In explaining the evolution of Medicaid, he notes that

> Mr. Wilbur Mills asked me what his answer would be to the inevitable question he thought he would be asked during the legislative debate: "Isn't Medicare an 'entering wedge' to a broader program of nationwide 'compulsory' insurance coverage of everyone?" I suggested that if he included some plan to cover the key groups of poor people, he would have a possible answer to this criticism. Medicaid evolved from this problem and discussion. I developed most of the provisions by expanding the plan requirements in the Kerr-Mills bill of 1960, taking into account the views of state welfare directors. Most federal and state public health officials had no interest in

administering such a program because of the fear that it would involve them in disputes with physicians. (P. 3)

In looking back over his forty-five years in government, Cohen saw "the Medicare and Medicaid legislation of 1965 as part of a long-term process—a continuation from the past, a creation in a particular moment of time, an incremental evolution for the future" (Cohen 1985:10).

The notion of national health insurance continued to percolate on the federal agenda throughout the optimistic years of the 1960s and into the 1970s. The issue during these years was less one of whether a national program was needed than its structure and operation. The debate, as was often common in the American context, was whether a new program should build on the existing private health insurance model or adopt a radical new approach involving the organization of a national health service with major planning and regulatory aspects. During these years unionized labor backed Senator Edward Kennedy's Health Security proposal based on a planning model, while the health industry and physicians supported an expansion of the existing system with federal assistance. By the early 1970s, the Nixon administration preferred a health insurance plan in contrast to simply expanding categorical entitlements and President Nixon endorsed national health insurance (Starr 1982). Senator Kennedy, seeing little support for his planning concept, joined Wilbur Mills in a proposal that shared many features with the administration's thinking and would use private insurers to administer the system. National health insurance seemed imminent. Ironically, organized labor, holding out for the original Kennedy concept, undercut the political momentum and their opposition resulted in a stalemate (Rivlin 1974). Changes in the economic fortunes of the nation, the persistently escalating costs of health care, growing concern about the federal deficit and American competitiveness, and antipathy to new taxes then pushed health insurance off the national agenda.

After a hiatus of more than fifteen years, universal health insurance is again an item on the social and political agenda. Although recession, the federal deficit, and concern about American competitiveness in world markets still encourage cautiousness in addressing the issue, the continuing uncontrollability of medical care costs, and the large size of the uninsured and underinsured populations, draw policy attention to the poor state of present arrangements and the need for reform. One major innovation is the growing tendency of some states to take the policy initiative and to develop approaches to extending insurance, regulating providers, and reallocating health expenditures (Aaron 1991).

The most immediate crisis in health care is the extraordinary segmentation of the health insurance marketplace, which has pushed large numbers of people outside the protective net of insurance. This reflects the historical tie of health care protection to employment; the changing character of the labor market, with the loss of numerous industrial jobs and the addition of poorly paid service jobs that offer less fringe benefits; and the continuing momentum of medical technology and health care costs, which increases the financial burden for employers. Hospitals have served the uninsured by shifting costs to other payers, but increasingly government and other payers have been restricting or protesting these transfers. Cost-shifting continues to drive premiums up, pushing many small employers and individual enrollees out of the health insurance market. These trends create considerable instability in insurance coverage, affecting far more people than is generally recognized. Twenty-eight percent of the population (more than 60 million people) did not have health insurance coverage for at least one month between February 1985 and August 1987 (Aaron 1991). The combination of influences described above results in an extraordinarily bizarre health care system that spends more and more money but disenfranchises a significant minority of the population.

In its early years, Blue Cross followed a philosophy of encouraging maximum community enrollment through rates that pooled risk across large segments of the public (Somers and Somers 1961). This concept of "community rating" encouraged insurance coverage for persons who otherwise might have become indigent patients if they became ill. This was attractive to the hospital sector and the concept worked exceedingly well when Blue Cross was the dominant insurer. In 1945 Blue Cross controlled 61 percent of the hospital insurance market, but by 1951 private commercial policies covered a majority of enrollees (Law 1974). Data reported by the Health Insurance Association of America (1990) indicates that Blue Cross-Blue Shield's share of the population of privately insured persons decreased from 47 percent in 1970 to 41 percent in 1988 (table 2.2). By the late 1950s it was clear that Blue Cross was losing the community rating battle, as commercial insurance attracted lower-risk persons at reduced premiums, requiring Blue Cross to increase its premiums to cover its more medically needy enrollees. By the 1970s, some Blue Cross plans were still trying to maintain the community rating ideal, fighting against the tide although losing the battle. In the 1980s, the Employee Retirement Income Security Act (ERISA), by exempting self-insured firms from state mandates for specified health benefits, encouraged self-insurance and further segmentation of risk (Fox and Schaffer 1989).

It is difficult to fault Blue Cross or employers for capitulating to a competitive ethos that destroyed health insurance as a community contract. In the early years, the social ideal served to expand the health insurance market and to support the growth of hospitals. It also weakened the case for national health insurance and, thus, received support from conservative interests (Stevens 1989:192). But it would be unrealistic to expect individual employers in a competitive economy to refrain from seeking to reduce their subsidies to the general population. Moreover, by the late 1970s the private insurance market had about reached its peak without additional forceful government intervention. Hospitals and various physician groups began to appreciate, following their experiences with Medicare, that national health insurance would probably be in their interest by providing payments for patients who are now the recipients of charity or subsidized care.

Although the development of the historical connection between employment and health insurance in the United States is easy to understand, it is increasingly a source of gaps in coverage. The largest gaps are found among low-paid workers in small businesses that fail to provide insurance, exclude coverage for dependents, or offer insurance at rates that many employees find prohibitive (Pepper Commission 1990). Insurance benefits are often nonportable, increasing discontinuity in coverage when workers move from one job to another or when they become unemployed. Students beyond their teens, often too old to be covered on parental policies but not yet in stable employment situations, also have a high risk of lacking insurance. Moreover, employer-based insurance creates a highly complex system with widely varying coverage among employees, and significant administrative costs.

One possibility for dealing with this situation, of course, is to significantly restructure the American health care system. It seems plausible that current spending of roughly $800 billion a year, and a projected $1.5 trillion by the year 2000 (Health Care Financing Administration 1987), should be sufficient to insure all Americans a reasonable level of health care, and much of this chapter addresses various aspects of this potential challenge. Yet, no one familiar with our health care system, and American politics, can fail to appreciate the obstacles to significant restructuring. Health care is now one of our largest social and economic sectors and a major source of employment and profit, and it serves many important and powerful interests exceptionally well. Thus, however enthusiastic we might be about planning yearly expenditures of $800 billion or a trillion dollars, there is little in the history of American social policy, in our political experience, or even in international endeavors that suggests that this is likely. This does not mean that we will not have substantial and meaningful change, only that we had better think very carefully about the structures that set the context for our future.

Politics generally involves a short frame of reference, usually bounded by the limited terms of office before public officials come up for election. A longer historical perspective suggests the possibility of major transformations in how we arrange our health affairs (Mechanic 1979; Starr 1982). Government support of managed care systems, prospective payment of hospitals, a resource-based relative-value scale for the payment of physicians, and many other increasingly accepted practices would have seemed subversive just a few decades ago. But the current concern with the federal budget deficit, and short-term perceptions of fiscal practicability, have encouraged even liberal forces to advocate relatively modest incremental improvements.

Bureaucracy and Administration

American medicine preserves the mirage of a private system at enormous administrative cost. Government directly pays for more than two-fifths of health care expenditures (Lazenby and Letsch 1990), and indirectly accounts for more through massive tax subsidies to businesses and individuals (Enthoven 1985). We create a large paper bureaucracy to maintain the illusion of free enterprise, but then regulate health providers more intensively and more intrusively than anywhere else in the world (Mechanic 1981).

Health care has become extraordinarily bureaucratized. As each new problem arises, and the problems are countless, government responds with additional regulatory requirements. In any given instance the requirements seem focused and responsive to the issues that motivated it, but in its totality the system is weighted down by massive and inconsistent requirements that put enormous drag on daily operations. Woolhandler and Himmelstein (1991) estimated that administration cost between $96.8 and $120.4 billion in 1987—19.3 to 24.1 percent of all expenditures. Between 1970 and 1982, while all health personnel increased by 57 percent, administrative personnel grew by 171 percent (Himmelstein and Woolhandler 1986). Administrative expenditures between 1983 and 1987 in constant dollars increased by 37 percent (Woolhandler and Himmelstein 1991). There is room to quibble about the size of these estimates, but no one who has even modest contact with the health sector can doubt the size, complexity, or burdens associated with the paper bureaucracy.

Simply dealing with billing and payment consumes enormous resources. Woolhandler and Himmelstein (1991) report that Blue Cross of Massachusetts employs 6,682 workers for an enrollee population of 2.7 million, more than the total administrators in Canada's health system covering 25 million people. Aggregated over the population, the time costs and frustration involved in processing multiple bills for many millions of episodes each year must be simply fantastic not only for the health system but also for patients who must cope with this complexity.

Public Perceptions of Our Health Care System

There is evidence of major dissatisfaction with the health care system. A recent Harris survey, for example, found only 10 percent of respondents agreeing that "On the whole the health system works pretty well, and only minor changes are necessary to make it better" (Blendon and Taylor 1989). In contrast, most respondents endorsed the need for fundamental change, and three-tenths thought that so much was wrong that we need to "completely rebuild it."

General attitudes however are not as informative as they may at first appear. Responses are substantially influenced by the wording and order of questions and the context in which they are asked. People are more likely to respond in less hypothetical situations in accord with personal interests than with overall impressions about social institutions and how well they work. Survey researchers have long recognized major incompatibilities between respondents' reports of general attitudes about health care and their own experiences (Andersen, Kravits, and Anderson 1971).

In surveys that address respondents' personal experiences there is typically considerable satisfaction expressed with one's personal physician
and treatment. Even in the Harris survey just noted, a majority of
respondents who used services were very satisfied with their physician
visits and hospitalization experiences, and only small minorities were
dissatisfied—13 percent for physician visits and 15 percent for hospital
care (Blendon and Taylor 1989). Other studies show even more profound
contradictions depending on wording of key items (Jajich-Toth and
Roper 1990, 1991).

There are a variety of hypotheses to explain the high degree of
personal satisfaction as reflections of the psychological need to report
satisfaction or of the fact that most people are reporting on their experiences when they are relatively healthy, and thus, deficiencies in care are
not salient. However, our efforts to focus attention in care surveys on
deficiencies or on populations who have the greatest needs for care have
not substantially increased the levels of reported personal dissatisfaction.

One suspects that the public's image of the deficiencies of our health
care system are shaped more by the mass media and the pronouncements
of experts than by their own experiences. Health care is a highly salient
theme for television, newspapers, and our national magazines, and
consumers are exposed to much expert criticism on uncontrollable costs,
the plight of the uninsured, the inadequacies of long-term care, excessive
profit-making and abuse, and the loss of caring practitioners. Health care
is seen by the media as in perpetual crisis, and all but the most oblivious
are aware of major problems.

The sources of discrepancies between general attitudes and personal
experiences thus emerge from conflicting channels of information. The
media emphasize the extraordinary cost escalation of medical care and
the public clearly recognize this as a major national problem. But in their
own experiences, most have insurance linked to their employment or the
employment of a family member and are insulated from high costs. In
many instances the insurance involves very small or no premium contributions, and while cost-sharing has increased in recent years (Gabel et
al. 1991), out-of-pocket expenditures for medical care for most of the
population remain modest relative to income. Household health spending
was 5.1 percent of adjusted personal income in 1989 (Levit et al. 1991),
an increase of 21 percent since 1965 but still within the modest range for
the average individual.

The difficulty is that not all people are average, and some face costs that are substantial. The media rightly emphasizes the plight of the uninsured, and surveys show considerable compassion for persons so affected. But the uninsured are a minority, and the problems of access to care they face do not touch most respondents in a personal way. In the abstract Americans abhor the fact that access to health care is determined as much by one's means as one's needs, and most are even willing to pay something more in taxes to remedy the problem. Few, however, are committed to pay the tax increases necessary within our current structure to provide universal access to those now disenfranchised. A 1990 survey found that 72 percent supported comprehensive national health insurance even when a tax increase was required, but only 22 percent were willing to pay more than $200 per year (Blendon and Donelan 1990). As in so many other areas in American life, the population quite readily endorses the goal but is resistent to making the sacrifices necessary (Etzioni 1991).

The discussion has given considerable attention to the issue of public opinion because, while we must be realistic about what public attitudes signify, the constellation of these attitudes provides a potential opportunity for future reform. The public shares an abstract predisposition toward restructuring, but one not strongly salient in affecting personal behavior or political engagement. A national leader who can effectively articulate the issues in an appealing way can draw on this general attitudinal resource to mobilize public opinion toward tangible political objectives. As gaps in insurance coverage affect larger numbers of people, opportunities increase for activating the population. This will not be easy, and the opposing political forces will be formidable, but the discomfort the public has about existing health arrangements presents a positive opportunity. It remains to be seen whether President Clinton can build the needed concensus to achieve the significant reforms needed and the nature of the compromises required.

Presidential leadership is extremely important and a major asset. Etheredge (1991) makes a good case, however, that the initiative for health policy reform has shifted to the Congress, and that momentum toward change is emerging through the reforms mandated in the Omnibus Budget Reconciliation Act of 1990, the establishment of commissions such as those on hospital and physician payment, and bipartisan efforts such as the Pepper Commission. Presidential involvement greatly enhances the potential, however, and President Clinton's commitment to health reform is a crucial ingredient in the emerging health landscape.

The Future: A Framework for Reform

Policy-making in health in the United States has become quite muddled about objectives. The "realists" have told us that planning is utopian, because politics and the powerful interests that have a large stake in the health economy will make such efforts irrelevant (Ginzberg 1977; Alford 1975). Thus, in the past decade we have focused on efforts to develop financial "fixes" that have diverted us from important priorities. The prevailing combination of free market rhetoric and intrusive regulation reflects confusion in our strategies and goals. Experts increasingly focus on smaller and smaller issues, not only separating the components from the overall objective but, even more important, doing so in a manner divorced from basic principles.

Although American medicine experimented with planning and regionalization at various points during the past twenty-five years, the planning process was typically given little power and was captured by the strong and aggressive provider community, doing little to insure a rational distribution and allocation of expensive resources. Planning, in a sense, became a "cost of doing business" that increased the costs of development and expansion without fundamentally altering its configuration. Thus, the planning process became one more layer of regulation.

American medicine, at this juncture, falls significantly short on each of the three basic goals that have guided health policy considerations over the past quarter-century—providing access in reasonable relationship to need; moderating the growth of medical care costs; and insuring uniformly high quality care. It has yet to give priority to expanding care so as to maintain function and quality of life not only for the elderly, but also for other populations having chronic diseases and significant disabilities. Extraordinary inequalities in health and health risks by race, class, and ethnicity persist, but care is distributed as much in relation to the ability to pay as it is to need. Prevention remains more rhetoric than reality, and rehabilitation principles, while highly developed in some specialized areas, have not yet entered the mainstream of care. There is much that is impressive in American medicine, but it is also evident that many of our citizens are outside the system and that we are far from realizing the value we should expect for the money we presently spend. The remainder of this chapter examines possible options for the future and barriers to their implementation.

Reform of our health system is a salient issue eliciting a large range of proposals (*Journal of the American Medical Association* 1991). Many proposals focus primarily on the uninsured population while others are aimed at restructuring the entire health care system. Blendon and Edwards (1991) have characterized these proposals as falling within four generic approaches. These include (1) requiring employers to provide private insurance with government filling the gap by providing insurance for those who are not employed; (2) giving employers the option of insuring their workers or alternatively paying a tax (the "play or pay" approach), with uninsured persons being covered by a government program as in the Massachusetts plan, and in a recent proposal by Senator Mitchell and other Democrats for health care reform; (3) using income-related tax credits to induce individuals to acquire private insurance along the lines proposed by Alan Enthoven; and (4) developing systems of national health insurance following such models as Canada or western European countries.

Despite the fact that health reform is again on the agenda, and there is much agreement on salient problems, all signs suggest little consensus about approaches to change and a protracted discussion. The outcomes will inevitably depend on the political process, and, thus, for my purposes here it is more useful to focus on some generic considerations than to spell out in detail my preferred solutions. I begin, however, with my own point of view since it helps the reader understand my perspective in examining other perhaps more politically viable alternatives.

The Canadian System

The Canadian system offers attractive features that would effectively address many of the problems we face. These include a federal-state system, universal and comprehensive coverage, portability between jobs and residence, reasonable access without copayment, nonprofit administration involving a single payor, negotiated budgets, and prospective hospital reimbursement. First as a federal-state system, with the federal government setting national standards and the states having a variety of implementation options, the Canadian approach fits our political structure and our preference for problem solving at the state level. The national standards of universal and comprehensive coverage would remedy the problems of instability of insurance tied to employment, underinsurance, and the problem of the uninsured. The standard of portability between jobs and residence would give individuals more freedom to choose jobs and geographic location independent of worry about maintaining health insurance. The implementation of nonprofit public administration of the system is likely to substantially reduce the claims bureaucracy, lessen burdens for physicians and patients, and save many billions of dollars. I also concur with the standard guaranteeing reasonable access without copayments and a prohibition on extra billing. As I will illustrate later, copayment reduces the demand for care, but not in a particularly rational way. Extra billing is unnecessary if physician payment is reasonable, which in all likelihood it would be in the American context.

In a recent report on Canadian health insurance, the General Accounting Office concluded that, "if the universal coverage and single-payer features of the Canadian system were applied in the United States, the savings in administrative costs alone would be more than enough to finance insurance coverage for the millions of Americans who are currently uninsured" (United States General Accounting Office 1991:3). The Accounting Office was particularly impressed by how the power of a single payer with authority to negotiate budgets, and the use of prospective budgeting of hospitals, were powerful instruments in successfully containing costs while providing all Canadians with reasonable access to primary care and generally appropriate services. Fixed prospective budgets are probably the only way we can ever gain control over medical care costs; the Canadian way is far more sensible and effective than the clumsy and overregulated incrementalism that characterizes our present path.

While I support a Canadian-type approach, there are several features that impress me as incompatible with American values and not particularly desirable in our context. In Canada, insurance companies are prohibited from selling insurance for services covered by the national plan, undermining any basis for a competing private system. Such a prohibition is consistent with a concept of equity and encourages, according to Hirschman's theory (Hirschman 1970), greater involvement in maintaining and improving the system, what he calls "voice" and "loyalty." A private competing system, in contrast, the theory suggests, encourages "exit" when people become dissatisfied, and thus less effort being put into improving the public arena. Certainly if the private system grows too large, these results are likely, but a modest private system complementing the public sector not only provides more choice and allows dissaffected and troublesome clients to go elsewhere but also serves as a comparison and challenge to the public system to maintain acceptable services. Thus, I support the concept of a parallel system. In contrast, I am sympathetic with prohibiting private practice among physicians working in the public system because dual practice risks encouraging two tiers within the same practice settings, but I anticipate that such a prohibition would not be acceptable.

The counterargument to the Canadian approach that will probably be a major concern for many Americans is that it strictly rations access to expensive technologies and treatments for patients except in emergency situations. Adequate data to assess this issue are not available and claims and interpretations tell you more about the ideologies of proponents than about the facts. In an effort to get more information, the GAO queried specialty directors in Ontario in charge of MRI, cardiovascular surgery, lithotripsy, and autologous bone marrow transplants. Questions referred to three types of cases, emergent, urgent, and elective. Respondents report substantial queues particularly for elective care, and sometimes the wait is very long (United States Government Accounting Office 1991:52-61). Considerable queuing was reported even for urgent cases defined as usually involving "serious medical conditions for which the patient is monitored and treated while in the hospital." It seems unlikely, given the high expectations of Americans, that they would accept rationing of technology of this magnitude, but following a Canadian approach does not imply a fixed level of access. Access must be structured, in part, in relation to the expectations and demands of the population. The challenge is to design a realistic structure for health care that operates within reasonable cost constraints but that is sufficiently flexible to respond to population demands and that is supportive of new opportunities to develop knowledge and technologies that significantly enhance the health of the population. The extent of rationing and queuing is ultimately a political decision.

Stating the challenge in such broad terms begs many questions because it is unclear how to define the value consensus, ascertain what expenditures are reasonable, or to determine which constraints will not stifle innovation and its applications. The health care industry is extraordinarily complex, involving thousands of interest groups highly protective of their domains. It is relatively easy to elicit agreement about abstract principles—for example that everyone should have access to needed health care or that everyone should have health insurance—but consensus breaks down quickly in considering concrete proposals that make the winners and losers apparent. This explains why efforts to improve systems of care almost always involve significantly increased expenditures, since cooperation and consensus are much more likely to be maintained when everyone involved has something to gain, as occurred in the implementation of the Medicare program.

There is widespread agreement that access to care when ill should be available; that primary care is needed to monitor health and illness in a continuing way; and that the health care system should give attention to prevention, health maintenance, and rehabilitation. The logic of primary care is that the provider takes continuing responsibility for monitoring health needs and is sufficiently linked into a larger network so that needed referrals are possible (Lewis, Fein, and Mechanic 1976). Primary care is an important enabling factor for appropriate referral and is not expensive relative to episodic outpatient hospital care typically found among disadvantaged patients. The Canadian system provides such care abundantly, using more physician services per capita than the United States (Fuchs and Hahn 1990). One short-term strategy for system reform would be to expand Medicaid or develop an alternative system to bring more of the disadvantaged into managed care systems emphasizing prevention, outreach services and continuity of care. Special efforts could be made to combine Medicaid with other entitlement programs to expand the range of traditional medical services responsive to patient need, including food supplements, assistance if necessary with housing problems, or help with other social problems.

This was the strategy when the Health Care Financing Administration launched a demonstration program on an expanded concept of care for the elderly—the Social Health Maintenance Organization (SHMO) (Greenberg et al. 1988). The goal is to integrate acute and necessary long-term care and to provide community-based care as an alternative to nursing homes. The services include homemaking, personal care, case management, adult day care and transportation, and patients are covered as well for a broader array of posthospital care than Medicare supports, including some custodial services. The four SHMOs that are part of this demonstration have been in operation for only four years and have had some start-up difficulties, particularly in the marketing and financial areas (Harrington and Newcomer 1991), but three of the four are now operating without deficits. This is a complicated but modest effort given the size and complexity of the health care system. We need much broader experimentation with extended care concepts as we begin to address long-term community treatment of serious chronic illness.

One such context is the care of seriously mentally ill persons in the community. As we have deinstitutionalized our public mental hospitals (Mechanic and Rochefort 1990), putting increasing reliance on general hospitals and other community facilities (Mechanic 1991b), we attempt to care for seriously ill patients with a broad array of psychiatric, medical, psychosocial, housing, and subsistence needs in the community. Care is highly fragmented. Efforts are now being made to integrate responsibility and fiscal authority to allow management of these broad needs within a single case-managed system using such devices as capitation and the development of public mental health authorities (Mechanic 1989a; Mechanic and Rochefort 1990). The need for integration of services is obvious in many other fields of chronic illness as well, including the care of persons with disabilities (Institute of Medicine 1991). Achieving this goal depends substantially on the enabling economic and organizational framework of care.

Alternative and Short-term Approaches to System Reform

Whatever the advantages of the Canadian model, it is more likely that reform will follow an incremental path by requiring or inducing employers to provide health insurance coverage for their workers and dependents. Through this process, varying gaps in coverage will be closed over time for insured workers, leaving smaller groups of uninsured to be covered by programs for the medically indigent. This could be accomplished by expanding eligibility under Medicaid or by developing alternative programs. Extending insurance coverage by itself doesn't address many of the problems already described, but it would contribute importantly to improving access to care.

A highly controversial approach is to extend coverage to a basic set of outpatient and inpatient benefits but exclude coverage of more discretionary services. This is what the state of Oregon has in mind in expanding eligibility for Medicaid benefits as a trade-off for a more restricted definition of the benefit package (Kitzhaber 1990; Eddy 1991; Dougherty 1991; Hadorn 1991). Although this is not a long-term solution, it is a plausible strategy as a stopgap measure during the stalemate over significant national reforms. The Oregon approach has been compromised practically and ethically, however, by exempting aged, blind and disabled recipients, thus putting the entire rationing burden on poor mothers and children who only account for about 30 percent of the Medicaid budget (Brown 1991). In principle, I am not in sympathy with those who oppose the Oregon and related approaches on the basis simply that they create two classes of care, although I find the selective exemptions disturbing. I prefer a single standard, but the alternative typically is no guaranteed care at all. The United States is a stratified society in almost every institutional sphere, and it is unlikely that we will see a single standard without a universal system. To oppose a rationing approach associated with increased eligibility because we aspire to a more comprehensive alternative is, in my view, not constructive.

Few challenge the notion of the guarantee of a basic minimum, but agreement on the boundaries of such an entitlement is difficult to achieve. While agreement may be possible on limitations of very high-cost but uncertain interventions such as the transplantation of hearts, lungs, or livers, the concept of what is basic depends substantially on a person's illness, disability, and level of function. Some argue, for example, that services for mental illness, alcohol abuse, and chemical dependency are discretionary, while persons with these problems see such services as central to their needs. Insurance for treatment of affective disorders and other mental illnesses, for example, is often limited (Mechanic 1989a), but depressive illness, and even depressive symptoms short of disorder, cause more pain, suffering, and disability than most common chronic medical conditions (Wells et al. 1989). Alternatively, one might choose to design benefits in terms of established knowledge of effectiveness (Brook 1991). Most widely used medical modalities, however, have never been rigorously evaluated, and establishing the needed research efforts is no small matter.

A major function of medical care is to provide reassurance, support, and health guidance. One strategy is to provide relatively easy access to primary medical care services, and associated cognitive services, within relatively lenient boundaries, but in systems in which primary practitioners have a gatekeeper role, as in the Canadian and British systems. Expensive modalities, in contrast, would be subjected to more rigorous tests of effectiveness, and access would be controlled. Thus, basic consultations concerning acute problems and health maintenance would be routinely available. As the costs of interventions increase, however, the evidential test justifying intervention and payment would be more explicitly established.

The Role of Competition

In recent years it has been argued frequently that many of the evident cost difficulties result from a lack of competition and absence of cost consciousness among consumers (Fuchs 1988). Competition is referred to in many ways, and the advocates often convey different conceptions.

One concept is that patients at the time of service should face sufficient cost-sharing so that they consider carefully the value of the service being sought. Coinsurance and deductibles are successful devices for reducing the demand for medical care and requiring consumers to pay more of the bill.

During the past decade much effort was made to shift costs back to patients. Justification for increased coinsurance came from the widely publicized findings of the RAND Health Insurance Experiment (Newhouse et al. 1981; Manning et al. 1988), which documented that coinsurance reduces the demand for ambulatory care. The prevalent economic theory posited that cost-sharing induced more careful and selective demand, thereby eliminating unnecessary and frivolous utilization. Later RAND analyses (Lohr et al. 1986), however, showing that cost-sharing inhibited demand in an unselective way, never achieved comparable visibility or attention. But the finding that cost-sharing did not result in appropriate selective decisions—that it inhibited efficacious as much as unnecessary care—points to the essence of the issue if the object of concern is the nation's health. Cost-sharing, a crude and irrational way to make allocation decisions, simply functions to reduce access and affects disproportionately those persons with the lowest incomes who have the highest needs for care.

Efforts at using economic incentives to induce cost consciousness among consumers are increasingly prevalent. But however much we try to objectify medical care, medical transactions in times of serious illness depend substantially on trust, and in any event, even the most motivated and sophisticated patients have difficulty obtaining the information necessary for independent critical judgments. Competition clearly has something to contribute in inducing consumers, when they are well, to choose carefully among competing health care plans. But knowledge about relative coverage and costs, the information typically available, reveals little about access to care, the quality of physician judgment, or physicians' commitment during a health crisis—issues extraordinarily difficult to obtain good information about (Mechanic 1989b). The essence of medicine to most people lies not in the services that are readily routinized but in the assurance that care will be of high quality when it counts, and that one's usual sources of care will mobilize intelligently when the circumstances warrant.

A more promising alternative, if we stay within our present framework of care, accepts the irrationality of asking sick people to assess the most cost-effective care option, and focuses on developing a system of managed competition in consumer selection among alternative health care plans. Enthoven's proposals (Enthoven 1980; Enthoven and Kronick 1989) for introducing a serious framework of managed competition among health care plans is theoretically persuasive, but achieving acceptance of the concept has been difficult in part because of the complexity of organization it requires. The basic idea is that people receive a health insurance subsidy sufficient to fund a basic health insurance policy that meets specified standards, to be selected from among a variety of competing plans. Employees choosing more expensive health insurance programs would have to bear the additional costs, and those selecting more economical options would be allowed to keep the savings. Competition at this level works but not as well as advocates suggest. There is an extraordinary degree of inertia among consumers and a strong preference to retain prior medical relationships if they are satisfactory (Mechanic 1989b). This explains the slow expansion of prepaid group practice in contrast to Preferred Provider Organizations (PPOs) that allow more choice. One would anticipate, however, that over time new cohorts would be socialized to receive their care in a managed care framework.

Managed competition will play some role in the future health care system but its form will depend on how our system evolves and political choices. We will return to a discussion of managed care, and some of the political choices involved, in chapter 10. Certainly if we continue with an employer-based insurance system, it would be constructive to offer patients meaningful choices and opportunities to save by selecting more economical health care options. If such a system is to avoid major deficiencies, the basic health insurance program should be adequate to meet critical health needs, and information about covered services and plan performance must be appropriate for making intelligent choices (Mechanic 1989b). In this sense, competition must be carefully regulated. Even if we were to go to a Canadian-type system, diversity and choice within the system would be helpful in shaping services toward consumer preferences, in contrast to bureaucratic inclinations.

Containing Costs

Expansion of coverage and enlarging the traditional goals of care to include promoting health must be linked to mechanisms that control overuse of expensive facilities, technical procedures, and professional services. Whether the United States could or should increase investments in health care to 15, 16, or even 20 percent of the gross national product is a political question and can only be resolved in that arena. In the absence of large new health investment, if we are to modify priorities—giving more emphasis to social and organizational technologies, education, and prevention—we must significantly restructure our ways of financing and organizing medical services. The inescapable conclusion—and one that has been with us for some time—is that we must have a controllable prospective budget and break away from reimbursement systems that pay for each service and procedure.

In the HMO model, the budget, based on capitation payments, sets constraints on expenditures and induces primary care physicians to be careful gatekeepers to the use of expensive modalities. In fee-for-service practice, similar constraints can be achieved through a fee schedule whose values are established in relation to total volume with a budgetary cap. Unlike a straight capitation that affects providers uniformly, the capped fee-for-service still allows individual physicians to increase their volume as much as they wish, but as physicians do this in the aggregate, each physician gets less per patient service. In the long run, any type of cap would do equally well in achieving cost constraint; but varying types of caps may have different consequences for how essential services are allocated and for professional morale (Mechanic and Faich 1970).*

The most simple constraint, and one likely to be more acceptable to professionals, is a fixed budget that sets a limit on total expenditures but does not specify the internal allocation of resources, leaving this to provider planning—a system of implicit rationing (Mechanic 1978b). Such an approach satisfies the payer's need to hold expenditures to a predetermined level without becoming involved in the thousands of decisions relevant to criteria for treatment and appropriate use of technology. An implicit rationing approach leaves these decisions to the managers and health professionals involved, honoring their professional and clinical autonomy. Government and other third parties are far removed from the pressures of illness and its complex contingencies and often introduce bureaucratic inflexibilities when they try to become involved in decisions at the micro level.

Implicit rationing, however, has some major weaknesses. It reinforces a highly discretionary system that can introduce considerable variability, responding differentially to patients by condition, social characteristics and personality. At the local level, professionals are much influenced by their prior training and personal experience and may make judgments that are less scientifically based than those made by a central authority that draws on the most rigorous research available. In any system of universal insurance, government has a stake in the principle that persons in comparable situations should be treated equally, but if each institution has discretion on how it uses available resources, major differences in access to treatment may result.

All systems are mixed, varying the balance between explicit directives and implicit processes (Mechanic 1979). Central decision making whether within a government authority or insurance program typically

---

* The current debate about implementation of the new physician payment arrangements under Medicare highlights the importance of building and institutionalizing trust. The medical community cooperated in developing these arrangements on the assumption that the payment system would be used to redistribute payment among procedures and specialties, but not to reduce the amount of payment. The Health Care Financing Administration, anticipating selective volume increases during the phase-in period has proposed cuts in fees to cover these costs. Physicians feel betrayed. HCFA may be technically correct, but has responded in a manner that violates prevalent understandings and undermines trust.

deals with issues such as the services covered, whether new experimental procedures and drugs should be covered, reimbursable providers, and related matters. The issue is how far-reaching explicit authority should be. In the case of highly expensive new technologies and eligibility or coverage rules, explicit authority is essential for establishing an equitable framework of care. It was fully reasonable for the Health Care Financing Administration to refuse to pay for tissue plasminogen activator (TPA), which cost far more than comparable drugs, when there was no evidence of its superiority. This action infuriated some physicians but it was a rational and appropriate decision (Mechanic 1989a). Much of the debate about central decision making focuses on the degree of micromanagement that is justifiable given the data capacities of central management and the variabilities in practice evident among physicians. My own view is that central management must be judicious and constrained, because it is likely to be insensitive to the complexity of medical transactions and the large variability in tastes, preferences, and orientations among patients. Physicians must retain considerable discretion, essential for subtle management of patients who often have complex diseases compounded by difficult social complications.

Essential to any fair system of implicit rationing is a budgeting process that is sensitive to the resource needs of each institution relative to the social and medical characteristics of the populations it is expected to serve. Payment to hospitals based on diagnostic-related groups is in essence a complexly stratified prospective payment plan that seeks to gauge payment in relationship to patient mix. Despite the detail involved, a persistent criticism of PPS is that the system is insufficiently sensitive to the severity of patient illness, particularly in institutions that serve large numbers of patients with medical problems compounded by socioeconomic disadvantage. Some efforts have been made to supplement payment to institutions that care for many indigent patients, but reimbursement practices are unlikely to address the true costs of a case-mix characterized by high proportions of disadvantaged patients.

The Question of Choice

As the United States has struggled with uncontrollable medical care costs, it has more aggressively supported the managed care approach and employers have more commonly adopted insurance programs that restrict consumer choice. Choice is important because it allows people to work out their different needs and tastes, and because people value services they personally select more than those imposed on them.

If the issue were simply satisfying people, and no more, a tough position based on conserving resources would be justified. Personal choice, however, is related to patient trust, cooperation in treatment, and response to treatment, and it contributes to keeping health professionals responsive. In clinical situations, the fact of choice acts as a placebo, enhancing the healing effect, because people are more likely to have faith in their provider and the decisions made. Beliefs can have a dramatic role in the illness process and substantially affect outcomes. They affect the amount of active participation individuals take in their own care—their conscientiousness in sharing vital information with their caretakers and in following prescribed regimens. Beliefs also are associated with a variety of biological responses to treatment, including the immune response, although the pathways of the process are still unknown. The evidence is persuasive that strongly felt beliefs can result in dramatic health improvement or, alternatively, in death (Frank and Frank 1991), and that people can affect the timing of their deaths, at least within short intervals (Phillips and Feldman 1973). A health care system, however scientific, that ignores beliefs and psychological realities loses much of its potential to care and possibly even to cure. The containment of aggressive technical care when it has marginal or no value is an immense challenge in the United States context. The American public highly values sophisticated technology, and the mass media are enthusiastic in their coverage of new treatment developments. Thus, consumer expectations and demands often reinforce physician predispositions and the financial and other incentives that influence their behavior. Different incentives would make it easier to shift these dispositions, but it is essential, too, that the public come to a better appreciation of the limits of medical intervention. This is an exercise in transforming our culture. It is hardly unusual that persons in pain, or those who are irreversibly ill or disabled, should hope to benefit from aggressive care or unproved therapies. We should support and sustain hope, of course, but doing so need not mandate the application of heroic interventionism that commonly exacerbates the miseries of serious and terminal illness. The growth of hospice care and of attention to living wills and power of attorney in health crisis situations suggests interest in alternatives among the general public.

A Framework for Reform: The Ideal and the Real

It is far too easy to construct a utopian health care system that has no possibility of implementation. The appealing logic of health systems with universal access, portability of health benefits, orderly relationships between primary, secondary, and tertiary care; broad concern with function and quality of life considerations as well as cure; and prudent expenditure patterns, requires no detailed explication. In fact, however, health systems never emerge anew, but are deeply embedded in the traditions, professional patterns, and organizational structures that have gone before and there is little reason to anticipate that future trends in American health care will be any different. Moreover, the size of the health care industry, and the magnitude of the vital interests of involved groups, makes straightforward reform extraordinarily difficult to achieve.

It would be helpful to eliminate employment-based insurance and develop a standard insurance program covering all eligible persons along the lines of the Medicare program or government-sponsored health insurance in other Western nations and Canada. The probability, however, is that we will not go this path, however reasonable. A significant proportion of the population is sufficiently content with their current source of insurance; very powerful interests have a stake in building on current mechanisms; and many fear the expected disruptions of moving to an entirely new approach. Thus, it seems likely that we will remedy gaps gradually through employer-mandated approaches, government-reated risk pools for the uninsured, and various possible extensions of Medicare and Medicaid. Some of these initiatives will develop through state legislation, but it seems inevitable that the federal government as well will have to engage these problems and provide assistance to states and small employers who are burdened by new insurance mandates. Over time, many of the known gaps will be closed but not without considerable waste and high administrative cost.

In the next decade, the focus will remain as much on cost as in the prior period. Although the Prospective Payment System reduced hospital expenditures to some degree below what they would have been without intervention (Russell 1989), government has been persistently unsuccessful in developing a viable approach to cost containment. The commonly used analogy of the balloon, which when pressed in one place bulges elsewhere, describes the situation. Although government has been making efforts over time to gain control over each practice sector, as it is now attempting in respect to physician payment, this remains a slow, awkward, and uncertain process. The provider community is extraordinarily creative in identifying loopholes, and we gain control over the system only with great administrative and regulatory cost. Our own history, and experience in other countries, suggests that we might be able to introduce a more streamlined national system if we were willing to spend lavishly, insuring that existing interests remain comfortable, but this alternative no longer seems feasible. Alternatively, approaching such major changes within an economically constrained framework is likely to encounter enormous resistance. While I hope for something better, I believe we will muddle along for years to come, trying one or another partial solution, and constructively filling some gaps. The world does change, and major dramatic innovations are not impossible. But in all likelihood, the future of health care reform is likely to be more a matter of incrementalism than a great leap forward.

The picture, however, is not entirely pessimistic. Any expanded view of the trajectory of health services will reveal some extraordinary changes in health services over the last several decades (Mechanic 1979). Medicare and Medicaid, while organized in an inefficient and costly way, dramatically changed the provision of health services and brought intensive, sophisticated care to many who never had such access before. These and other federal programs stimulated a health infrastructure and technological capacity that is truly impressive. We have a large and well-trained corps of health professionals who have a capacity to serve our population exceedingly well. In some sense, what we lack most is a sense of discipline and fairness in capitalizing on this capability. Our problem, thus, resides not with our basic assets but rather with both the excesses and the deficiencies of their utilization. The challenge is one of organization and our political capacity to bring a greater sense of prudence, balance, and equity to how we manage our health affairs.

References

Aaron, H.J. 1991. *Serious and Unstable Condition: Financing America's Health Care*. Washington, DC: The Brookings Institution.
Alford, R. 1975. *Health Care Politics: Ideological and Interest Group Barriers to Reform*. Chicago: University of Chicago Press.

Andersen, R., Kravits, J., and Anderson, O.W. 1971. "The public's view of the crisis in medical care: An impetus for change in delivery systems?" *Economics and Business Bulletin* 24:44-52.

Assistant Secretary for Health. 1990. *Healthy People: National Health Promotion and Disease Prevention Objectives.* DHHS Pub. No. (PHS) 91-50213. Washington, DC: U.S. Government Printing Office.

_____. 1979. *Healthy People: The Surgeon General's Report of Health Promotion and Disease Prevention.* DHEW (PHS) Pub. No. 79/55071. Washington, DC: U.S. Government Printing Office.

Ball, R.M., and Bethell, T.N. 1989. *Because We're All In This Together.* Washington, DC: Families U.S.A. Foundation.

Blendon, R.J., and Donelan, K. 1990. "The public and the emerging debate over national health insurance." *New England Journal of Medicine* 323:208-12.

Blendon, R.J., and Edwards, J.N. 1991. "Caring for the uninsured: Choices for reform." *Journal of the American Medical Association* 265:2563-65.

Blendon, R.J., and Taylor, H. 1989. "Views on health care: Public opinion in three nations." *Health Affairs* 8:149-57.

Brook, R. 1991. "Health, health insurance, and the uninsured." *Journal of the American Medical Association* 265:2998-3000.

Brown, L.D. 1991. "The national politics of Oregon's rationing plan" *Health Affairs* 10:28-51.

Bunker, J.P., Gomby, D.S., and Kehrer, B.H. 1989. *Pathways to Health: The Role of Social Factors.* Menlo Park, CA: Henry J. Kaiser Family Foundation.

Chassin, M.R., Kosecoff, J., Park, R.E., Winslow, C.M., Kahn, K.L., Merrick, N.J., Keesey, J., Fink, A., Solomon, D.H., and Brook, R.H. 1987. "Does inappropriate use explain geographic variations in the use of health care services: A study of three procedures." *Journal of the American Medical Association* 258:2533-37.

Cherlin, A.J., Furstenberg, F.F. Jr., Chase-Lansdale, P.L., Kiernan, K.E., Robins, P.K., Morrison, D.R., and Teitler, J.O. 1991. "Longitudinal studies of the effects of divorce on children in Great Britain and the United States." *Science* 252:1386-89.

Cohen, W.J. 1985. "Reflections on the enactment of Medicare and Medicaid." *Health Care Financing Review,* 1985 Annual Supplement, 3-11.

Dougherty, C.J. 1991. "Setting health care priorities: Oregon's next steps. A Conference Report" *Hastings Center Report* 21:1-11.

Dubos, R. 1959. *Mirage of Health.* New York: Harper & Brothers.

Dutton, D.B. 1986. "Social class, health, and illness." In Aiken L.H. and Mechanic, D. (eds.), *Applications of Social Science to Clinical Medicine and Health Policy.* New Brunswick, NJ: Rutgers University Press, 31-62.

Eddy, D. 1991. "What's going on in Oregon?" *Journal of the American Medical Association* 266:417-20.

Eisenberg, J. 1991. "Economics." *Journal of the American Medical Association* 265:3113-15.

Enthoven, A. 1985. "Health tax policy mismatch." *Health Affairs* 4:5-14.

_____. 1980. *Health Plan: The Only Practical Solution to the Cost of Medical Care*. Reading, MA: Addison-Wesley.

Enthoven, A., and Kronick, R. 1989. "A consumer choice health plan for the 1990s." *New England Journal of Medicine* 320:29-37, 94-101.

Etheredge, L. 1991. "Negotiating national health insurance." *Journal of Health Politics, Policy and Law* 16:157-67.

Etzioni, A. 1991. "Too many rights, too few responsibilities." *Society* 28:41-48.

Fox, D.M. 1986. *Health Policies, Health Politics: The British and American Experience 1911-1965*. Princeton: Princeton University Press.

Fox, D.M., and Schaffer, DC 1989. "Health policy and ERISA: Interest groups and semipreemption." *Journal of Health Politics, Policy and Law* 14:239-60.

Frank, J.D., and Frank, J.B. 1991. *Persuasion and Healing*, 3d ed. New York: Schocken Books.

Freeman, H., Kiecolt, K.J., and Allen, H.M.II. 1982. "Community health centers: An initiative of enduring quality." *The Milbank Quarterly* 60:245-67.

Fuchs, V. 1988. "The 'competition revolution' in health care." *Health Affairs* 7:5-24.

_____. 1968. "The growing demand for medical care." *New England Journal of Medicine* 279:190-95.

Fuchs, V., and Hahn, J.S. 1990. "How does Canada do it?: A comparison of expenditures for physicians' services in the United States and Canada." *New England Journal of Medicine* 323:884-90.

Gabel, J., DiCarlo, S., Sullivan, C., and Rice, T. 1991. "Employer-sponsored health insurance, 1989." *Health Affairs* 9:161-75.

Geiger, J. 1984. "Community health centers: Health care as an instrument of social change." In Sidel, V.W. and Sidel, R. (eds.), *Reforming Medicine's Lessons of the Last Quarter Century*. New York: Pantheon.

Ginzberg, E. 1977. *The Limits of Health Reform: The Search for Realism*. New York: Basic Books.

Glaser, W.A. 1970. *Paying the Doctor*. Baltimore: Johns Hopkins University Press.

Greenberg, J., Leutz, W., Greenlick, M., Malone, J., Erwin, S., and Kodner, D. 1988. "The social HMO demonstration: Early experience." *Health Affairs* 7:66-79.

Hadley, J., Steinberg, E.P., and Feder, J. 1991. "Comparison of uninsured and privately insured hospital patients: Condition on admission, resource use and outcome." *Journal of the American Medical Association* 265:374-79.

Hadorn, DC 1991. "The Oregon priority-setting exercise: Quality of life and public policy." *Hastings Center Report* 21:11-16.

Harrington, C., and Newcomer, R.J. 1991. "Social Health Maintenance Organizations' service use and costs, 1985-89." *Health Care Financing Review* 12:37-52.

48   Inescapable Decisions

Health Care Financing Administration. 1987. "National health expenditures, 1986–2000." *Health Care Financing Review* 8:1–36.
Health Insurance Association of America. 1990. *Source Book of Health Insurance Data*. Washington, DC: HIAA.
Himmelstein, D.U., and Woolhandler, S. 1986. "Cost without benefit: Administrative waste in U.S. Health Care." *New England Journal of Medicine* 314:441–46.
Hirschman, A.O. 1970. *Exit, Voice, and Loyalty: Responses to Declines in Firms, Organizations, and States."* Cambridge: Harvard University Press.
Hsiao, W., Braun, P., Dunn, D. Becker, E.R., Denicola, M., and Ketcham, T. 1988. "Policy implications of the resource-based relative value study." *New England Journal of Medicine* 319:881–88.
Institute of Medicine. 1991. *Disability in America: Toward a National Agenda for Prevention*. Washington, DC: National Academy Press.
Jajich-Toth, C., and Roper, B.W. 1991. "Basing policy on survey data: Proceed with caution." *Health Affairs* 10:170–72.
_____. 1990. "Americans' views on health care: A study in contradictions." *Health Affairs* 9:149–57.
Journal of the American Medical Association. 1991. Special Edition: "Caring for the uninsured and underinsured." Vol. 265, no. 19.
Kark, S.L., and Steuart, A. 1962. *A Practice of Social Medicine*. Edinburgh: ETS Livingstone.
Kemper, P., Applebaum, R., and Harrigan, M. 1987. "Community care demonstrations: What have we learned?" *Health Care Financing Review* 12:37–52.
Kitzhaber, J.A. 1990. "The Oregon model." In *The Richard and Linda Rosenthal Lectures*. Washington, DC: Institute of Medicine, 69–80.
Law, S. 1974. *Blue Cross: What Went Wrong?* New Haven: Yale University Press.
Lazenby, H.C., and Letsch, S.W. 1990. "National health expenditures, 1989." *Health Care Financing Review* 12:1–26.
Leventhal, H. Prohaska, T.R., and Hirschman, R.S. 1985. "Preventive health behavior across the life span." In Rosen, J.C., and Solomon, L.J.(eds.), *Prevention in Health Psychology*. Hanover: University Press of New England, 191–235.
Levit, K.R., Lazenby, H.C., Letsch, S.W., and Cowan, C.A. 1991. "National health care spending, 1989." *Health Affairs* 10:117–30.
Lewis, C.E., Fein, R., and Mechanic, D. 1976. *A Right to Health: The Problem of Access to Primary Medical Care*. New York: Wiley-Interscience.
Lohr, K.N., Brook, R.H., Kamberg, C.J., Goldberg, A., Leibowitz, A., Keesey, J., Reboussin, D., and Newhouse, J.P. 1986. *Use of Medical Care in the Rand Health Insurance Experiment: Diagnosis- and Service-Specific Analyses in a Randomized Controlled Trial.* Publication No. R-3469-HHS. Santa Monica, CA: RAND Corporation.

Luft, H. 1987. *Health Maintenance Organizations: Dimensions of Performance.* New Brunswick, NJ: Transaction Publishers.

Manning, W.G., Newhouse, J.P., Duan, N., Keeler, E., Benjamin, B., Leibowitz, A., Marquis, M.S., and Zwanziger, J. 1988. *Health Insurance and the Demand for Medical Care.* RAND Health Insurance Experiment Series. Santa Monica, CA: RAND Corporation.

Marmor, T.R. 1973. *The Politics of Medicare.* Chicago: Aldine.

McCord, C., and Freeman, H.P. 1990. "Excess mortality in Harlem." *New England Journal of Medicine* 322:173-77.

Mechanic, D. 1991a. "Strategies for health promotion." Proceedings of the Second International Conference of Health Behavior Sciences, Tokyo, Japan, Japan Academy for Health Behavioral Research.

_____. 1991b. "Recent developments in mental health: Perspectives and services." *Annual Review of Public Health* 12:1-15.

_____. 1990. "Promoting health." *Society* 27:16-22.

_____. 1989a. *Mental Health and Social Policy,* 3d ed. Englewood Cliffs, NJ: Prentice-Hall.

_____. 1989b. "Consumer choice among health insurance options." *Health Affairs* 8:138-48.

_____. 1981. "Some dilemmas in health care policy" *The Milbank Quarterly* 59:1-15.

_____. 1979. *Future Issues in Health Care: Social Policy and the Rationing of Medical Services.* New York: Free Press.

_____. 1978a. *Medical Sociology,* 2d ed. New York: Free Press.

_____. 1978b. "Approaches to controlling the costs of medical care: Short-range and long-range alternatives." *New England Journal of Medicine* 298:249-54.

_____. 1974. "Patient behavior and the organization of medical care." In Tancredi, L.R. (ed.), *Ethics of Health Care.* Washington, DC: Institute of Medicine, National Academy of Sciences, 67-85.

Mechanic, D., and Aiken, L.H. 1991. "Caring and the structure of health care services." Paper presented at the Conference on the Caring Physician. Center for Advanced Study in the Behavioral Sciences, Palo Alto, CA.

_____. 1989. "Access to health care and use of medical care services." In Freeman, H., and Levine, S. (eds.), *Handbook of Medical Sociology,* 4th ed. Englewood Cliffs, NJ: Prentice-Hall.

Mechanic, D., Ettel, T., and Davis, D. 1990. "Choosing among health insurance options: A study of new employees." *Inquiry* 27:14-23.

Mechanic, D., and Faich, R. 1970. "Doctors in revolt: The crisis in the national health service." *Medical Care* 8:442-55.

Mechanic, D., and Rochefort, D. 1990. "Deinstitutionalization: An appraisal of reform." *Annual Review of Sociology* 16:301-27.

National Center for Health Statistics. 1991. *Health, United States, 1990.* Hyattsville, MD: Public Health Service.

Newhouse, J.P., Manning, W.G., Morris, C.N., Orr, L.L., Duan, N., Keeler, E.B., Leibowitz, A., Marquis, K.H., Marquis, M.S., Phelps, C.E., and Brook, R.H., 1981. "Some interim results from a controlled trial of cost sharing in health insurance." *New England Journal of Medicine* 305:1501–507.

Office of National Cost Estimates. 1990. "National health expenditures, 1988." *Health Care Financing Review* 11:1–54.

Office of Technology Assessment. 1987. *Neonatal Intensive Care for Low Birth Weight Infants: Costs and Effectiveness.* Publication No. OTA–HCS–38. Washington, DC: U.S. Government Printing Office.

———. 1985. *Technology and Aging in America.* Publication No. OTA–BA–264. Washington, DC: U.S. Government Printing Office

Pauly, M.V. 1988. "Review of 'Caring for the Disabled Elderly'." *Health Affairs* 7:169–72.

Payer, L. 1988. *Medicine and Culture: Varieties of Treatment in the United States, England, West Germany, and France.* New York: Henry Holt.

Pepper Commission. 1990. *A Call for Action: Final Report of the U.S. Bipartisan Commission on Comprehensive Health Care.* Washington, DC: U.S. Government Printing Office.

Phillips, D., and Feldman, K. 1973. "A dip in deaths before ceremonial occasions: Some new relationships between social integration and mortality." *American Sociological Review* 38:678–96.

Report of the Secretary's Task Force on Black and Minority Health. 1985. Washington, DC: U.S. Government Printing Office.

Rice, D., and Feldman, J. 1983. "Living longer in the United States: Demographic changes and health needs of the elderly." *The Milbank Quarterly* 61:362–96.

Rivlin, A.M. 1974, 21 July. "Agreed: Here comes national health insurance." *New York Times Magazine*, p. 8.

Rivlin, A.M., and Wiener, J.M. 1988. *Caring for the Disabled Elderly: Who Will Pay?* Washington, DC: The Brookings Institution.

Robert Wood Johnson Foundation. 1991. *Environment for Learning.* An Interim Report of the Robert Wood Johnson Commission on Medical Education: The Sciences of Medical Practice. Princeton, NJ: Robert Wood Johnson Foundation.

Russell, L.B. 1989. *Medicare's New Hospital Payment System: Is It Working?* Washington, DC: Brookings Institution.

———. 1986. *Is Prevention Better than Cure?* Washington, DC: The Brookings Institution.

Russell, M.A.H., Stapleton, J.A., Jackson, P.H., Hajek, P., and Belcher. 1987. "District programme to reduce smoking: Effect of clinic supported brief intervention by general practitioners." *British Medical Journal* 295:1240–44.

Russell, M.A.H., Wilson, C., Taylor, D., and Baker, C.D. 1979. "Effect of general practitioners' advice against smoking." *British Medical Journal* 2:231–35.

Shy, K.K., Larson, E.B., and Luthy, D.A. 1987. "Evaluating a new technology: The effectiveness of electronic fetal heart rate monitoring." *Annual Review of Public Health* 8:169–90.

Shy, K.K, Luthy, D.A., Bennett, F.C., Whitfield, M., Larson, E.B., van Belle, G., Hughes, J.P., Wilson, J.A., and Stenchever, M.A. 1990. "Effects of electronic fetal-heart-rate monitoring, as compared with periodic auscultation, on the neurologic development of premature infants." *New England Journal of Medicine* 322:588–93.

Somers, A.R. 1987. "Insurance for long-term care: Some definitions, problems, and guidelines for action." *New England Journal of Medicine* 317:23–29.

Somers, H.M., and Somers, A.R. 1961. *Doctors, Patients, and Health Insurance.* Garden City, NY: Anchor-Doubleday.

Starr, P. 1982. *The Social Transformation of American Medicine.* New York: Basic Books.

Stevens, R. 1989. *In Sickness and In Wealth: American Hospitals in the Twentieth Century.* New York: Basic Books.

Svarstad, B. 1986. "Patient-practitioner relationships and compliance with prescribed medical regimens." In Aiken, L.H. and Mechanic, D. (eds.), *Applications of Social Science to Clinical Medicine and Health Policy.* New Brunswick: Rutgers University Press, 438–59.

Tennstedt, S.L., and McKinlay, J.B. 1989. "Informal care for frail older persons." In Ory, M.G., and Bond, K. (eds.), *Aging and Health Care: Social Science and Policy Perspectives.* London: Routledge.

Thomas, L. 1977. "On the science and technology of medicine." *Daedalus* 106:35–46.

United States General Accounting Office. 1991. *Canadian Health Insurance: Lessons for the United States.* Publication No. GAO/HRD-91-90. Washington, DC: U.S. Government Accounting Office.

Waitzkin, H. 1983. *The Second Sickness: Contradictions of Capitalist Health Care.* New York: Free Press.

_____. 1979. "A Marxist interpretation of the growth and development of coronary care technology." *American Journal of Public Health* 69:1260–68.

Waitzkin, H., and Britt, T. 1989. "Changing the structure of medical discourse: Implications of cross-national comparisons." *Journal of Health and Social Behavior* 30:436–49.

Warner, K.E., 1987. "Health and economic implications of a tobacco-free society." *Journal of the American Medical Association* 258:2080–86.

Weissert, W.G. 1991. "A new policy agenda for home care." *Health Affairs* 10:67–77.

Wells, K.B., Stewart, A., Hays, R.D., Burnam, A., Rogers, W., Daniels, M., Berry, M.S., Greenfield, S., and Ware, J. 1989. "The functioning and well-being of depressed patients: Results from the Medical Outcomes Study." *Journal of the American Medical Association* 262:914–19.

Woolhandler, S., and Himmelstein, D.U. 1991. "The deteriorating administrative efficiency of the U.S. health care system." *New England Journal of Medicine* 324:1253-58.

2

Sources of Countervailing Power in Medicine

A growing literature is directed to the corporatization of medicine, to the loss of physician autonomy, and to the alleged deprofessionalization and proletarianization of doctors (McKinlay 1988). These concepts relate to a number of long-standing debates among sociologists concerning the character of the professions and the evolution of capitalist society and engage especially those with Marxist proclivities. I largely sidestep these arguments because I believe that focusing on whether doctors are as professional as they once were, or are being proletarianized, is not to the point. Following Willie Sutton, who explained that he robbed banks because that's where the money was, I would rather focus my attention on the integrity of emerging health care organization and its responsiveness to the needs of the population than on whether physicians perceive a loss of autonomy.

The theory of proletarianization, as McKinlay and Stoeckle (1990) describe it, "seeks to explain the process by which an occupational category is divested of control over certain prerogatives relating to the location, content, and essentiality of its task activities, thereby subordinating it to the broader requirements of production under advanced capitalism" (p. 144). The authors define seven areas in which professional prerogatives of physicians have eroded: defining entrance criteria for becoming a physician; deciding the terms and content of their work; their relationships to clients; technology; facilities; and the amount and rate of their remuneration. McKinlay and Stoeckle's documentation on these points tends to be general and ambiguous. For example, in respect to medical school admissions, they note that the schools are "forced to" recruit minorities and women, and on curriculum they observe that government and other interests affect content through training programs, student loans, and the like. One might argue that the authors are stretching their argument with such weak examples. All social institutions are expected to increase participation of minorities and women, and government programs and incentives affect behavior across institutions of every kind. These authors, recognizing that their evidence is less than persuasive, qualify their case by noting that proletarianization is "a useful explanation of a process under development, not a state that has been or is just about to be achieved."

McKinlay and Stoeckle explicitly link proletarianization to corporatization, a process they define only with examples of the growth of corporate entities in the health field. Their Marxist explanation of change is that investors need to rationalize production and that, as a result, physicians lose traditional professional prerogatives. As Roemer (1986) has suggested, a more politically neutral account of corporatization is necessary. It would help counter the charge leveled in so much of the corporatization literature that this type of organization is inherently exploitative. The types of organizations emerging in health include not-for-profit as well as profit chains and religious as well as secular organizations. There is little doubt that bureaucratization is increasing (Mechanic 1976), but its causes and consequences are not self-evident. Navarro (1988), from a different perspective, is critical of the confusion between corporatization and proletarianization. He acknowledges that physician autonomy has eroded but challenges the notion that physicians and their professional representatives are likely to relate to the working class in mind or action.

Current debates about physician autonomy and proletarianization look very different when considered in the context of the changing nature of medical institutions and their roles in the broader economy. The model of the individual physician as an entrepreneurial professional, free to define the character of his or her work and how to perform it (Freidson 1970a 1970b), has diminishing relevance given an increasingly sophisticated technological superstructure, and at a time when biomedical knowledge is rapidly advancing and professional decisions translate into enormous expenditures of other people's money, whether government or private.

The escalation of medical care costs in the United States and other Western countries draws intense scrutiny on medicine. National health expenditures in the United States have grown from 4.4 percent of gross national product in 1955 to 12 percent today. While a similar trend exists throughout the developed world, nowhere has medicine's share of national wealth escalated so rapidly, or consumed so much on a national or per capita basis. The extent to which health expenditures create profitable markets, compete with other national needs, and put pressures on governmental and private-sector budgets helps explain the attention and increasing intrusions on the practice of medicine. Technological developments, demands for equity of access, and an aging population all entail the possibility of expanding costs. As long as some see little reason why the proportion of gross national product for health should not go to 15 percent or higher, it is no surprise that government, industry, and the public at large are prepared for regulatory initiatives that would have seemed inconceivable a decade ago.

My thesis is that the perception of growing encroachment on the physician's autonomy reflects less the erosion of an earlier demarcated turf than the transformation of medical practice following World War II, particularly in the past several decades, into what is now a major sector of our national economy. Concomitantly, the physician has evolved from a "bit player" who for most of history has struggled as an individual entrepreneur to eke out a good living from patients willing to pay fees—often with hardship—into a decision maker who could order the expenditure of other people's money in large sums.

In calling the pre-World War II physicians "bit players," I don't mean to suggest that they lacked power, prestige, admiration and considerable social influence. Physicians in both the pre- and postwar period had a strong sense of self-efficacy and political legitimacy, were highly admired by the general population as numerous studies show, and had large influence on medical social policy. Eliot Freidson's description (1970a, 1970b) of their dominance is typical. But it wasn't until late in the 1960s that medicine emerged as a major sector of our economy, consuming ever larger proportions of our gross national product, federal and state expenditures, and industrial fringe benefits. It has been estimated that each physician, in addition to his or her own income, accounts for expenditures in the range of $500,000 to $800,000 a year. In the case of the most technologically sophisticated specialties, the figure may well be in the millions. Playing on this larger turf involves new rules and many more of them, and appropriately so.

With the growth of health insurance and the erosion of the direct link between services given and payments received, doctors make claims on insurance companies and government budgets in a manner not easily controlled. The extension of insurance not only increased the demand for care but also loosened the constraints on how physicians used expensive resources, since neither patient nor doctor perceived anything to lose and sometimes both saw something to gain. Advanced forms of regulation thus emerged in which payment involves third parties, not just those engaged in the medical transaction, and in which the potential costs are high. While it is true that regulatory efforts are easier to administer in hospitals than in doctors' offices, and in surgery than in general medicine, the main focus on hospitals and surgery is due more to the dollars involved than to ease of administration.

The Growth of Countervailing Power

In the pre-World War II years, government and business had less stake in how physicians carried out their work than they do now. Individual patients cared deeply, since they were often digging into their own pockets to pay the required fees, and exercised some client control (Freidson 1970a). The growth of third-party insurance following the war was encouraged by the hospitals that were seeking new paying clients, and in those days bills were paid with little second-guessing (Law 1974). The notion of challenging physician decisions was novel, and in any case, conflict would have interfered with the growth of insurance, which had broad support. But now the stakes are higher, and challenges to health sector decisions have become politically more necessary and acceptable.

Physicians would have us believe that they are rapidly losing control over the conditions of their work. Some outside observers, in contrast, see the inability to control costs as a product of an unequal contest between a relatively united medical profession and large numbers of unaffiliated payers (Reinhardt 1989). A major factor differentiating the United States from such other nations as Canada, West Germany, and Sweden in the ability to constrain rising medical costs is the way potentially countervailing agencies are organized. In most nations with systems of national health insurance, the price of care is established in negotiations between government or large sickness funds with physicians as a group (Glaser 1970), a process not lacking acrimony but one in which the forces are more equally balanced than in the United States. In the United States, in contrast, the multiplicity of payers makes it relatively easy for physicians to reject patients when their insurers refuse to meet price demands (as in the Medicaid program), and the fragmentation among payers gives physicians considerable leverage in establishing their fees. If there was one payer or a limited number of them, physicians would be less able to set the terms of their own remuneration.

Since many physicians increasingly depend on Medicare payments for a significant proportion of their remuneration, the Health Care Financing Administration (HCFA), acting under Congress's direction, has considerable countervailing power in establishing physicians' fees. Until now, HCFA has had little authority over fees, but as we move into an era of resource-based relative-value scales and expenditure targets, it seems inevitable that government will be a tougher adversary in fee-setting consistent with the types of constraints introduced by the Prospective Payment System for hospitals. Government may seem too tough or too lenient, depending on where one sits, but the size of Medicare as a payer increasingly balances the contest. The magnitude of government's investment gives it opportunity to influence doctors' decisions in a wide variety of ways.

Doctors can still locate niches that allow traditional practice without much external intrusion but such potential opportunities are diminishing and cannot support large numbers of an increasing corps of physicians. Modern practice, in most advanced specialties, is highly interdependent and requires a level of capital expenditure for necessary equipment and facilities that fewer physicians than before can manage on their own. Even the practice of independent physicians coming together to capitalize expensive technology—a pattern of traditional organization astutely managed by private entrepreneurial physicians—is constrained by the size of the investments required, making it possible for venture capital such as in for-profit companies to compete successfully with independent physicians. Given the billions of dollars of potential profit, and the assortment of new coalitions competing for such profits, many new types of alliances have emerged.

As the necessity to manage this large public expenditure for medicine becomes evident, the variability in expensive practices becomes more salient and the need for national standards more obvious. Most of what physicians do depends more on professional experience and judgment than on well-established knowledge justifying one course of action over another. Their decisions are not easily controlled at the level of clinical management, but they can be more readily monitored in their use of discrete procedures, such as specific surgical interventions or diagnostic modalities. Although more uncertain, controls can also be applied by defining ranges of appropriate treatment such as length of hospital stay or classes of appropriate medication. It is now part of conventional wisdom that much of medical care lacks demonstrated efficacy, although estimates of the magnitude of ineffective practice seem to vary widely. One sophisticated physician estimates that no more than 15 percent of medical procedures have been suitably established to be efficacious (White 1988), and there are increasing numbers of studies showing the high rate of procedures that fail to meet even loose standards of appropriateness (Chassin et al. 1987).

There is much agreement that existing incentives encourage over-utilization of expensive and dangerous modalities, but there is a disconcerting lack of interest in the larger epidemiological picture and the extent to which useful modalities are not provided to persons who could benefit. It has long been known that physician decisions vary across regions and small geographic areas, but increasingly, studies of practice variations have brought these large variations to the consciousness of policymakers and the public. Since the procedures under consideration are expensive, and many involve risks of iatrogenic illnesses as well, there is strong interest in bringing them within more limited bounds. Implementation still depends largely on educational efforts, but formal protocols for many of these procedures are being developed, and their imposition through regulation appears inevitable in the future. The use of such protocols will, without doubt, restrict the discretion of the individual doctor, as the algorithms used by professional review organizations sometimes do now. Such protocols may be seen as interfering with the individual clinician's autonomy but it should be noted that they are the product of medical research and physician judgment. Thus, they reflect the bureaucratization of peer physician regulation, but at a national rather than a local level.

The centralization of bureaucratic authority in HCFA and in state regulatory agencies is understandably frightening to many physicians. The average physician has become dependent on revenues from the Medicare program as have hospitals, nursing homes, and other providers. HCFA is developing a national data file as a basis for a program of studies on effectiveness of medical procedures, and this effort is intended to serve as guidance for reimbursement policy. The new agency on health care policy and research will also focus on medical effectiveness reinforcing trends toward greater standardization. Physicians are now required to provide diagnostic codes on each bill submitted, and other coding expectations will inevitably follow. The ultimate capacity to track the work of each physician over time gives what some see as awesome future powers to HCFA.

HCFA, however, is not unconstrained. Its influence is shaped by the political process, and by the pressures brought by various interest groups on the federal executive and the Congress. One of the weaknesses of our federal system is the fragmentation of authority and the difficulty of forming a consensus around tough reforms in which there will be significant and powerful losers. The process induces compromise and HCFA is not immune. There is, however, concern in the professional community that HCFA not develop the instruments that would allow it to "tighten the screws" at times when those outside the profession strengthen their political will. The professional community understands that once the mechanism to exercise tighter controls is in place, it is more likely to be used, particularly as the saga of uncontrollable costs continues.

Physician Response

Even the most cursory examination of medical practice and the roles and authority of physicians across nations reveals how deeply they are embodied in the history of each nation and its cultural experience. The traditional stratification of physicians in any country and their unique relationships to government and other sectors typically have deep foundations. I focus exclusively on the American situation, where the data are better, but, even here, the existing literature gives insufficient attention to the heterogeneity of physician roles, the variations among varying cohorts of physicians, the complexity of the internal stratification of doctors, and the networks of influence that affect health policy.

To physicians in midcareer, the conditions of practice and the complexity of reimbursement and other practice arrangements appear to have changed dramatically. Public expectations have increased, demanding both technical excellence and competence in a broad range of functions ranging from preventive behavior modification and sex counseling to cost-effective practice behavior. Patients appear more demanding and critical, and the rising cost of malpractice insurance and threat of malpractice litigation add a sense of anxiety to what was already in doctors minds a feeling of general bewilderment. Insurance intermediaries, after a long history of passivity, have begun to question claims more aggressively, and professional review organizations, unlike earlier professional standards review organizations, are somewhat tougher watchdogs. The freedom of physicians to bill as they wish will persist only if they are confident enough to opt out of major health entitlement programs as few are, given the growing dependence of their incomes on such programs. And the practice of extra-billing in the Medicare program faces increasing restrictions and possibly ultimate prohibition. The perceived threat to their professional authority is exemplified by nurses employed by professional review organizations informing physicians that a decision to hospitalize a patient is unjustified. Nurses in these situations are not independent decision makers applying a medical algorithm to admission and discharge decisions. Symbolically, however, the nurse telling the doctor that he or she can't hospitalize a patient represents a reversal of everything that older doctors have learned to take for granted.

What strikes older physicians as representing a conversion of their world may have less poignancy to those just entering medicine who are socialized into new forms of bureaucratic practice and who, thus, experience much less discontinuity in their practice worlds. While concerned about their economic prospects, they are less likely to experience as indignities third-party involvement or changing roles and responsibilities among varying health professions. But the issue is less what doctors feel and more what the impact is of changing rules and organizational configurations on their practice behavior. And, here, the younger doctors are perhaps more affected than those further along in their careers because they have yet to develop a practice and are more likely to enter group practices and HMOs where their professional life is more bureaucratized.

Although physicians in group practice have always experienced some difficulties in accommodating their personal preferences to the demands of a group organization, those in prepaid practice, in particular, are increasingly exposed to administrative pressures. Most basic are the increasingly forceful incentives to conserve resources through fewer hospital admissions and surgical interventions and careful ordering of tests and procedures. HMOs commonly both withhold payment and provide bonuses as incentives for careful expenditure patterns. Hillman (1987) was able to obtain information in 1987 from about half of the active HMOs on a list maintained by InterStudy. Two-thirds of all HMOs reporting withhold a portion of payments to primary care physicians, usually in the range of 11 to 20 percent. For-profit HMOs were more likely to withhold: 70 percent of them withhold compared to 58 percent among not-for-profits. Thirty percent of HMOs, in addition, put primary care physicians at risk of additional financial penalties. A more important issue is the extent to which the primary physician should be held at *personal* financial risk for high expenditures or whether the risk should be divided among an entire group of physicians. Eighteen percent of HMOs put physicians at risk for personal performance; such mechanisms, however, are far more common in for-profit HMO plans (23 percent among for-profit, compared with 9 percent among not-for-profit). Hillman and his colleagues found that putting physicians personally at financial risk and imposing additional penalties for deficits beyond the amounts withheld resulted in fewer outpatient visits per enrollee. As far as I can ascertain, this is the only study that has examined the consequences of putting physicians at personal risk. It should be obvious that much more information is necessary on the consequences of these and other types of efforts to balance the role of physician as the patient's agent against his or her role as allocator of limited resources.

A recent analysis of data from a 1987 survey of young physicians (defined as less than forty years old, and between two and six years beyond graduate training) (Hadley et al. 1990) helps us understand how current trends affect persons early in their careers. Approximately one-third of the respondents indicated that if they were doing it over again they would not go to medical school; but a realistic assessment of this response would be difficult. Jack Hadley and his associates (1990) used a logistic regression technique to examine factors associated with physicians' "second thoughts" and the wish to change the current way they practice. Controlling for sociodemographic variables, type of medical school, and years in practice, those most likely to have second thoughts reported significantly lower incomes (both per hour and on an annual net basis), higher educational debt, and more work effort, especially during nights and weekends. Thus, those doctors who felt that their economic return was low relative to their investment and income were more likely to have second thoughts.

An analysis by Willke and associates (1990) of employment arrangements of young physicians using the same data set shows continued strong momentum in early careers toward self-employment. In the second year of practice, 42 percent of young physicians are already self-employed, mainly in solo or small practice groups. Among those in the fifth year of practice, 59 percent are self-employed. Employed physicians, thus, remain in the minority and experience more personal constraints. Hadley and his associates, for example, found that employed physicians who had "second thoughts" compared to those who did not, reported significantly more often that they didn't have the freedom to spend sufficient time with patients, to carefully review patients' medical histories and test results, to hospitalize patients they felt required it, to control their own work schedule, to order tests and procedures whenever they wanted, and to care for patients unable to pay the fees and charges. Unfortunately, comparable questions could not be asked of self-employed physicians. One should note, however, that employed physicians seldom reported constraints on freedom. Less than one-tenth reported lack of freedom to hospitalize patients and care for patients who couldn't pay, and only 14 percent reported a lack of freedom to order tests and procedures whenever they wanted.

The largest constraints reported by employed physicians were a lack of freedom to control their own work schedule (43 percent) and their inability to spend sufficient time with patients (23 percent). In theory, self-employed physicians are free to do as they wish, but as other studies show they also feel severe time and scheduling constraints (Mechanic 1975a). These problems are exacerbated in highly organized group practice, in which most employed doctors find themselves, but they are generally characteristic of all medical practice in which demand is high and reimbursement is tied to physician productivity. The difference is that self-employed physicians are economically rewarded for each increment of effort while employed physicians see less connection between their work efforts and economic rewards (Mechanic 1974, 1975a).

The evidence is slim that physicians, whatever they fear or believe, are losing their clinical autonomy. Their feelings of loss are probably provoked by a sense that the amount of effort they expend is no longer tied to the payments they receive. As salary and capitation become more prevalent types of payment, such perceptions are likely to increase, unless the remuneration is very generous. The evidence is persuasive that money is the crux of the issue. If the payment is sufficiently large, physicians appear satisfied whatever its form. An exception is when it is anticipated that the payment mechanism will be used to reduce future remuneration. The Willke study (1990) of young physicians for the American Medical Association helps us understand that the key to satisfaction and dissatisfaction among young physicians is still substantially a matter of personal economic interest and the relative degree to which payment is consistent with personal expectations and the degree of effort expended (see also Hadley et al. 1990).

Implications of Current Trends

There have been major changes in the organization, financing, and culture of medicine in the past quarter century. Thus, it seems reasonable to assess how fundamental these changes are for the role and status of the medical practitioner. Are doctors becoming deprofessionalized and proletarianized, as some claim? Or do the observed changes reflect more the changing science and technology of medical work and the emergence of better educated and more sophisticated populations and increased demands for equal access?

There is little doubt that modern medical practice is increasingly corporatized, if one means by this simply that it is organized within more complex organizational forms, characterized by corporate objectives and some division of responsibility between management and operations (Fried, Deber, and Leatt 1990). If this were the only issue, there would be little room for discussion or controversy. The controversy comes not from basic disagreement about these facts but more from the implications by many who write about the topic that the trend is evil and exploitative (see Salmon 1990). Here I side with Milton Roemer (1986), who views the emerging social organization of health care as a trend toward more effective health services, "mediated largely (though not entirely) through political processes" (p. 469). The influence of emerging trends on the status of physicians as professionals needs examination on at least three levels—what I here refer to as the cultural, social, and personal.

At the cultural level, I would argue that there has been enormous expansion in the importance of medicine and the public's perceived dependence on it. Although there are occasional examples of issues that have been redefined to fall outside traditional medical domains—for example in the assessment of homosexuality—the major impetus has been toward a growing medicalization of personal and social problems (Zola 1983). There seems little that does not fit within expanding medical boundaries, and despite some strong protests from women's groups and persons with disabilities, these expansions have received considerable political and cultural legitimacy. American society has an almost insatiable interest in health and medical affairs, one that some of our foreign friends view as obsessive. The mass media track every potential biomedical advance, and the well-informed public regularly learns of the latest research published in the *New England Journal of Medicine* and the *Journal of the American Medical Association* often well before their physicians read about it. We need serious scholarly inquiry of these seemingly important cultural changes but, for our purposes here, it seems clear that medicine as a cultural enterprise has lost no ground in recent decades.

Similarly, despite much rhetoric, there is little evidence that the social place of medicine or its intellectual dominance has eroded. Almost all of the changes characterizing the emerging social organization of medical practice are fully consistent with dominant medical perspectives; indeed, these changes are, in part, responses to imperatives of new medical knowledge and technologies (Mechanic 1975b). Social historians remind us that there are alternative ways of organizing around any technology and no single mode of organization is predetermined (Stevens 1989; Rosenberg 1987; Starr 1982). The organizational developments that we see in medicine may not, therefore, be the only ones possible, but they do mesh with the complex technologies that have emerged from advances in biomedical science.

Cost containment in medicine occupies much attention in political discussions, the media, and the profession. It is easy to overlook the modesty of cost-containment goals—simply reduce the rate of increase and not challenge in any fundamental way whether the medical model is worthy of the enormous societal investment it receives. The value of such investments is not in any sense obvious when one considers the opportunities forgone in equal or more important social priorities. Some analysts discuss the issue from time to time, but it's hardly a question taken seriously in decision-making circles. The recent call for effectiveness research itself reflects the traditional standard of scientific medicine to demonstrate the clinical value of its modalities. Nowhere in the vast array of changes that have affected medicine in recent years, or among the new nonmedical participants in health policy, can one find any serious challenge to the hegemony of the medical perspective.

This is not to suggest either that the personal power and autonomy of the individual physician has not weakened or that there has been an absence of counterchallenges to the biomedical imperative. But neither of these trends has gone as far as many predicted. Insofar as physicians are affected, medicine has retained its economic and technical control to an extraordinary degree despite conditions that might have substantially undermined the profession's power base. The growing supply of physicians and the heterogeneity of their background and interests have not had the anticipated impact on fees and remuneration that market models might predict. Although physician income in constant dollars has lagged in recent years, the profession continues to maintain very high incomes, a mean net income of $155,800 in 1989. A few years ago, some were predicting the emergence of a few national "super-meds," firms that would come to control most of the medical care marketplace. Not only has this not occurred but, in addition, for-profit corporate ventures have suffered serious economic setbacks. While there was much talk of large for-profit firms dictating the conditions of medical practice, much of their efforts have focused on cost, hardly an unreasonable concern given the financial context of health care.

Perspectives that compete with the medical model are only dimly perceived, in part because medicine has been so successful in dominating the public's conception of health and disease. Medicine is ecumenically organized and has had an almost infinite capacity to absorb competing perspectives without any significant change in course. The UCLA Medical School can hire Norman Cousins to lecture on holistic health concepts while pursuing its emphasis on high-technology biomedical research; doctors can talk about a new emphasis on prevention; and medical journals can abundantly report the need for a long-term care perspective and a new biopsychosocial model, emphasizing care rather than cure. But as Deep Throat advised, "Follow the money." And if we do so, we find a system of care heavily weighted to high-technology curative care in contrast to the promotion of function and quality of life (Mechanic 1989). At the social level, we see a system that is patient—not population—based, with glaring inequities in access to health insurance and basic health care. However much medicine appears to have changed, and however many the forces buffeting it, its traditional pathways and resilience seem as strong as ever.

The forces arrayed against medicine perhaps lead us to exaggerate their significance. Other health professions have not seriously challenged physicians' dominance, although a few have found marginal niches where they exercise relative independence (professional psychology and nurse practitioners). For-profit medicine has introduced constraints but has not fundamentally changed the ways doctors work. The evidence shows no large differences between profit and non-profit institutions (Gray 1991). Indeed, many profit institutions make special efforts to win over the somewhat skeptical physician community and are very responsive the their perceived needs. Patients may be better educated than ever before, and some more demanding, but most still remain docile. Pressures from women have modified obstetrical practices and a variety of social amenities, but if one looks a bit deeper the trend is steadily toward caesarean deliveries, more electronic fetal monitoring, and the increased medicalization of the natural process of childbirth (Mechanic 1989). Moreover, when outside parties have intruded on medical work, it has typically been justified by reference to physician experts and the extant medical literature.

This is not to imply that physicians have no cause for anxiety. Government has been putting into place the tools necessary to regulate medical care much more closely and in finer detail than ever before. The significance of diagnosis-related groups and expenditure targets is not so much that they contain costs to some degree, but that they ultimately become the mechanisms that allow payers to control the flow of public expenditures. All such systems begin generously, but they typically rachet down prices when economic conditions require it.

What government can do depends on political acceptability. As long as physicians retain the respect and loyalty of the public, they have considerable influence to contain countervailing forces. As public disillusionment grows, government gains more confidence in its ability to intercede. But the chips in the game are still largely medical and represent the alternative visions of physicians on how to define and deliver effective health care.

References

Chassin, M.R., Kosecoff, J., Park, R.E., Winslow, C.M., Kahn, K.L., Merrick, N.J., Keesey, J., Fink, A., Solomon, D.H., and Brook, R.H. 1987. "Does inappropriate use explain geographic variations in the use of health care services: A study of three procedures." *Journal of the American Medical Association* 258:2533-37.

Freidson, E. 1970a. *Profession of Medicine: A Study of the Sociology of Applied Knowledge.* New York: Dodd Mead.

_____. 1970b. *Professional Dominance: The Social Structure of Medical Care.* New York: Atherton.

Fried, B.J., Deber, R.B., and Leatt, P. 1990. "Corporatization and deprivatization of health services in Canada." In Salmon, J.W. (ed.), *The Corporate Transformation of Health Care: Issues and Directions.* Amityville, NY: Baywood Publishing Co., 167-86.

Glaser, W.A. 1970. *Paying the Doctor.* Baltimore: Johns Hopkins Press.

Gray, B. 1991. *The Changing Accountability of Doctors and Hospitals.* Cambridge: Harvard University Press.

Hadley, J., Cantor, J.C., Kidder, S., Willke, R.J., Feder, J., and Cohen, A.B. 1990. "Second thoughts about becoming a physician: Evidence from a survey of young physicians." Unpublished paper. Washington, DC: Center for Health Policy Studies.

Hillman, A. 1987. "Financial incentives for physicians in HMOs: Is there a conflict of interest?" *New England Journal of Medicine* 317:1743-48.

Law, S.A. 1974. *Blue Cross: What Went Wrong?* New Haven: Yale University Press.

McKinlay, J.B. (ed.). 1988. "The changing character of the medical profession." *The Milbank Quarterly* 66:supp. 2.

McKinlay, J.B., and Stoeckle, J.D. 1990. "Corporatization and the social transformation of doctoring." In Salmon, J.W. (ed.), *The Corporate Transformation of Health Care: Issues and Directions.* Amityville, NY: Baywood Publishing Co.

Mechanic, D. 1989. *Painful Choices: Essays on Health Care.* New Brunswick, NJ: Transaction Publishers.

_____. 1976. *The Growth of Bureaucratic Medicine.* New York: John Wiley.

_____. 1975a. "The organization of medical practice and practice orientations among physicians in prepaid and nonprepaid primary care settings." *Medical Care* 13:189-204.

_____. 1975b. "Ideology, medical technology, and health care organization in modern nations." *American Journal of Public Health* 65:241-47.

_____. 1974. "Patient behavior and the organization of medical care." In Trance024, L.R. (ed.), *Ethics of Health Care.* Washington, DC: Institute of Medicine, National Academy of Sciences, 67-85.

Navarro, V. 1988. "Professional dominance or proletarianization?: Neither." *The Milbank Quarterly* 66:57-75.

Reinhardt, U.E. 1989. "The U.S. health care financing and delivery system: Its experience and lessons for other nations." Paper delivered at the International Symposium on Health Care Systems, Taipei, Taiwan.

Roemer, M.I. 1986. "Proletarianization of physicians or organization of health services?" *International Journal of Health Services* 16:469–71.

Rosenberg, C. 1987. *The Care of Strangers: The Rise of America's Hospital System.* New York: Basic Books.

Salmon, J.W. (ed.), 1990. *The Corporate Transformation of Health Care: Issues and Directions.* Amityville, NY: Baywood Publishing.

Starr, P. 1982. *The Social Transformation of American Medicine.* New York: Basic Books.

Stevens, R. 1989. *In Sickness and in Wealth: American Hospitals in the Twentieth Century.* New York: Basic Books.

White, K. 1988. Foreword. In Payer, L., *Medicine and Culture: Varieties of Treatment in the United States, England, West Germany, and France.* New York: Henry Holt.

Willke, R.J., Marder, W.D., Kletke, P.R., Emmons, D.W., Loft, J.D., and White, M.L.S. 1990. "Early professional development in medical practice." Unpublished paper. Chicago: American Medical Association, Division of Survey and Data Resources.

Zola, I.K. 1983. *Socio-Medical Inquiries.* Philadelphia: Temple University Press, 247–68.

3

Professional Judgment and the Rationing of Medical Care

The Context of the Rationing Debate

As medical care costs in the United States escalate and account for a growing proportion of gross national product, health care rationing, once commonly viewed as unthinkable, has become an increasingly respectable response. The popular conception of rationing is based on the American experience of food and gasoline rationing during World War II, in which specified shares of a limited resource were distributed. Fixation on such an extreme example obscures the fact that substantial rationing occurs every day in the distribution of the limited resources of all publicly supported services (Friedman 1971). This de facto rationing is so common in everyday reality that it is hardly thought of as rationing at all.

The lack of awareness of hidden subsidies and funding limits is not unique to the health care rationing situation but describes much of the intersection between marketplace and social policy. Most middle-class Americans fail to recognize the extensive subsidies they receive for health care, housing, and other services. Thus, they perceive that housing subsidies are solely given to the poor, failing to recognize the much larger housing subsidies to the middle class through the opportunities to deduct interest for home loans on their tax return. Alain Enthoven (1985) estimated that revenue loss in 1985 resulting from favorable tax treatment of employer contributions for medical insurance and medical care was approximately $47 billion.

Background of Rationing

Throughout most of medical history, the availability of medical services was substantially rationed by the ability to pay, by the availability of number and types of practitioners and facilities in different geographic areas, and by patient compatibility with physicians' research needs and practice inclinations (Mechanic 1979). To the extent that the market for medical care was primarily private, the ability of people to pay for medical care set strict constraints on its consumption. Although many physicians provided considerable charity care to patients who lacked resources, financial concerns constrained the extent of such charity efforts.

The growth of health insurance and large government programs—particularly Medicare and Medicaid—in the post World War II period has fundamentally changed health care utilization by separating the patient's ability to pay from the availability of medical services. Once one gains eligibility or pays health insurance premiums, the received entitlements are only tangentially related to out-of-pocket expenditures, if at all. This change has weakened the influence of economic constraints on patient behavior, skewing the consumption of certain medical services.

Currently, rationing occurs mostly through the design of health insurance coverage and reimbursable providers, rather than by the patient's ability to pay. Individual and administrative choices are made among coverage options for competing service benefits, types of facilities and practitioners, and contexts of care, including hospitals, nursing homes, outpatient settings, and the home. Initially, most insurance covered hospital care and only a limited scope of possible health care needs. While these insurance programs expanded, they generally continued to limit coverage in such areas as mental health, dentistry, outpatient prescription drugs, and podiatry. For instance, less than half of the elderly's health care costs are covered by Medicare despite the magnitude of Medicare expenditures as a percentage of national health care expenditures.

Rationing also results from how care is organized. The structural organization of medical care has inherent imbalances, such as the unequal availability and distribution of tertiary care facilities, specialized hospitals, nursing homes, outpatient programs, rehabilitation facilities, and various types of reimbursable practitioners. These imbalances limit the services available to persons in some geographic areas. Such constraints are further reinforced in most insurance programs by cost-sharing, through co-insurance and deductibles, limits on the frequency and intervals within which certain services can be utilized, and maximum allowable expenditures on various types of benefits.

These methods of rationing had been obscured by the rapid growth of health insurance and health expenditures during the post-World War II period. Financial incentives created by Medicare reimbursement and tax policies stimulated the expansion of hospitals and development of new nursing homes. The number of nursing home beds, for example, grew from fewer than 570,000 in 1963 to approximately 1.4 million by 1976. As medical knowledge and new technologies expanded, public expectations of the quality of health care increased. Because most people had greater access to care than previously, and certainly more than earlier generations, access inequalities and limitations on the services available were not generally recognized. Moreover, because insurance mechanisms were separate from the supply of facilities, programs, and practitioners, the public did not see an obvious link between the theoretical availability of entitlements and difficulties in obtaining them. Despite the public's ignorance, rationing was in fact occurring.

New medical care financing made available by Medicare, Medicaid, and other government programs altered the supply of services. These programs were biased toward the reimbursement of technical procedures, in contrast to providing cognitive and counseling services characteristic of primary care. Large inequalities in access persisted by geography, urban or rural residence, and the demographic characteristics of varying population groups. Thus, resource limitations moderated the pace of growth, but not to the extent of requiring "tragic choices" (Calabresi 1974).

Today the need for rationing is clear. Medical expenditures have escalated dramatically since federal Medicare and Medicaid programs were initiated in 1965, and they will continue to grow due to rapid advances in science and technology, a growing population of elderly with a high prevalence of chronic disease, increasing patient expectations, and an expanding population of health professionals and physicians who to some degree create demand for their own services. The crux of the current debate is not whether we should ration care. Rather, having recognized that rationing is inevitable, the debate focuses on the appropriate mix of rationing devices to constrain supply and allocate it fairly, in a manner consistent with an acceptable quality of care.

This debate does not exist in a vacuum; health care in the United States is a public endeavor to a significant degree. The government, in some form, directly pays for more than 40 percent of all health care costs and an even larger proportion of the costs for inpatient care and the uses of expensive technology (Lazenby and Letsch 1989). Through its tax and reimbursement policies, the government substantially subsidizes the purchase of health insurance and the capacity of nonprofit and private institutions. Future health care reforms may require employers to provide health insurance to their workers, a form of indirect taxation. Thus, government has a large and growing stake in the shaping of future constraints and an examination of possible approaches to rationing becomes necessary.

Approaches to Rationing

One alternative strategy to rationing health care is to increase the proportion of the cost paid by the patient, thus reducing the cost borne by government (price rationing). With the emphasis on competition during the 1980s, substantial increases in cost-sharing were introduced across the entire health care sector. One obvious advantage of price rationing is that it reduces the financial burden on government or insurer by requiring patients to share an increased part of the cost. Additionally, price rationing is motivated by the theoretical belief that if individuals are required to pay part of the costs of their medical care, they will consider the need for care more carefully and choose services more selectively, thus reducing trivial and inappropriate demands for care. General support for this proposition comes not only from economic theory, but also from early results of the RAND Health Insurance Experiment (HIE), which demonstrated that copayment significantly reduced the demand for ambulatory care (Newhouse et al. 1981). Subsequent research from the HIE found that copayors did not differentiate between appropriate and inappropriate care (Lohr et al. 1986; Siu et al. 1986). Thus, one could conclude that copayment reduced demand for care, but not in a discriminating or rational way. Copayment also deters the poor from seeking care to a greater extent than the affluent, even though poverty is associated with more illness and a greater need for care.

The second alternative strategy for rationing health care is through explicit legislative mandates and administrative decisions. Such explicit constraints are common and include definitions of eligibility for program enrollment, decisions about the services and procedures to be reimbursed, criteria defining eligibility for specified services, and definitions of reimbursable providers and eligible location of service provision. When explicit rationing is used, regulators may describe in detail the services that will be available and the criteria for their allocation and monitor care processes by preliminary review, second opinions, and audits to assure that clinicians follow specified algorithms. Explicit rationing also refers to procedures limiting the expansion of facilities, such as certificates of need, regulations concerning the acquisition and use of technology, and budgeting decisions constraining the development and diffusion of technologies. Limitations of technical capacity and facilities results in queuing, a pervasive and effective rationing approach.

One advantage of explicit rationing is that a central authority can develop sophisticated data systems and appraisals of the scientific literature to inform those making funding decisions about technologies and services. The central authority can draw on high levels of scientific and professional expertise and can synthesize large quantities of pertinent data. Such a centralized authority, properly staffed, can make more scientifically sophisticated choices than individual professionals who proceed on the basis of a fragmentary command of scientific evidence and who are strongly influenced by their personal clinical experience.

Significant progress is being made, using complex multivariate techniques, in analyzing clinical data to predict therapy outcomes for critically ill patients (Knaus et al. 1991). Some of these models predict more accurately than experienced clinicians, and pressures will increase to use such systems and constrain physician decision making. As these new techniques become more sophisticated, they will be powerful aids in medical assessment, but are unlikely to substitute for an individual professional's judgment. As William Knaus and his colleagues note,

Physicians have also been hesitant to apply probability estimates to a particular patient. The physician always knows elements of the patient's condition that are not in the predictive model, and rarely is there evidence to show that the additional information is irrelevant. Knowledgeable physicians are also concerned over whether current patients and treatments are truly comparable to those in the predictive model and whether the identical therapies were used for patients in the database. (P. 390)

Clearly, central authority must set broad constraints on the definition of reimbursable services and technologies if costs are to be constrained in our world of limitless possibilities. Detailed rule making, however, is too distant from the realistic contingencies of disease, the complexities of comorbidity, and the diversity of personal and family situations to extend to specific clinical decisions under the conditions of uncertainty that characterize much of medical care. In a large and culturally heterogeneous society it is especially difficult to anticipate the varying needs, expectations, and tastes of patients and their families, and the varying and shifting family structures and social situations that are pertinent to the choices people make and their effective care.

This leads to the third alternative, implicit rationing, in which regulatory authorities set general constraints on expenditures, entitlements, and expensive technologies, but the actual allocation of services is determined within doctor/patient transactions. The English National Health Service, the Canadian Medicare System, and HMOs in the United States reflect implicit rationing to some extent. Despite information problems, implicit rationing at the level of the individual physician within broad constraints is the best option. Because a strong relationship often develops between doctor and patient in critical illness situations, resulting in a high level of trust and a high quality of communication between them, the individual physician is in the best position to make good health provision judgments. The disadvantage of implicit rationing is that it may erode trust between the doctor and patient by assigning the doctor a dual responsibility of choosing between an individual patient and other patients' priorities. While troublesome, this disadvantage is more palatable than the lack of understanding and insensitivity likely to result from explicit rationing decisions made in a micromanagement mode by persons removed from the complicated situations and emotions associated with illness and the help-seeking process.

The Case for Implicit Rationing

The Substance of Medical Care

Implicit rationing, despite some obvious limitations, offers the best opportunity to allocate care effectively in the context of uncertainty, a changing knowledge base, and heterogeneity in the American population and in patterns of illness.

In the typical medical encounter the patient presents a variety of complaints to a physician who, by selectively questioning the patient, seeks to identify an underlying pattern and to diagnose it. The diagnosis operates as a working hypothesis, suggesting varying degrees of information about the etiology and course of the problem as well as approaches to treatment. If the patient's problem is clear, and fits a well-established diagnostic theory, then the diagnosis itself offers a prescription for how the physician should proceed in specific treatment and overall care management (Mechanic 1978).

The difficulty is that many problems do not allow clear diagnostic determinations, or are complicated by comorbid conditions. Often the treatment plan is uncertain because preferred modalities are not supported by clear scientific evidence. Kerr White, a distinguished observer of the medical care process, observed that "it is still the case that only about 15 percent of all contemporary clinical interventions are supported by scientific evidence that they do more good than harm" (White 1988). Numerous studies document extraordinary variabilities in practice. There are also high levels of inappropriate use of technologies as evaluated by implicit medical criteria. Confusion exists, however, because of the difficulty of documenting any substantial relationship between practice variation and inappropriate applications (Chassin et al. 1987; Leape et al. 1990).

Substantial literature documenting enormous geographical variations in the performance of discretionary procedures suggests that high rates of utilization are associated with unnecessary and inappropriate care. If prevalence is associated with an unnecessary or inappropriate pattern of care, constraining the trend by regulation would be feasible. However, the reality is far more complex, less well understood, and more imposing from a regulatory perspective. Two RAND studies of utilization of coronary angiography, carotid endarterectomy, and gastrointestinal tract endoscopy by Medicare beneficiaries in small area aggregations found little relationship between the prevalence of these procedures and their appropriate use as measured by a careful evaluation of medical records based on carefully formulated criteria (Chassin et al. 1987; Leape et al. 1990). There was, in fact, enormous variation in the use of these procedures. The investigators identified care that they rated as inappropriate, but there was no obvious explanation for these differences. It is therefore difficult to understand how we can impose intelligent, explicit rationing when we cannot clearly isolate the factors that account for existing practice variation.

The mismatch between the magnitude of variation and definitions of appropriateness reflects practices under conditions of uncertainty (Eddy 1984), which must be accepted until firmer knowledge is available. The lack of precision in medical care judgments makes offering directives that cover the entire range of clinical alternatives a risky proposition. Either more conservative or more radical treatment alternatives can be advocated; the scientific evidence does not support a clear choice. Most physicians can agree that computerized automated tomographic (CAT) scans, nuclear magnetic resonance (NMR) imaging, and other expensive diagnostic modalities are used excessively. It may, however, be impossible to specify all of the contingencies that would distinguish justifiable from unjustifiable use.

No reasonable way exists of addressing this challenge within the confines of explicit rationing. Writing detailed specifications will encumber clinicians in an extensive web of regulations that will result in many ambiguities, difficulties, and absurdities. Moreover, a necessarily changing knowledge base requires continuing modifications—a source of regulatory chaos. Currently prevailing incentives encourage the use of resources on the margin because technical procedures are remunerative for the physician and involve little out-of-pocket expense for the patient. Explicit rationing that limits the capacity for expensive diagnostic and treatment modalities through some form of regional scheme could be a solution. The queue for treatment would then serve to limit demand by restricting supply. Queuing, however, which is based on a first come, first served principle, does not distinguish between those patients who have a higher than average probability of benefiting from the intervention and those who are "lost causes." Once again, some level of professional judgment is essential to allocate available resources in relation to need and expected benefits.

Individual physicians could reasonably exercise such judgment if constrained by the knowledge that the pool of resources available for the care of their patients is finite, and that indiscriminate or careless use would limit valued diagnostic and treatment possibilities for others. Such implicit rationing is common in most public institutions throughout our society, including schools, social services, the courts, and almost all other public and nonprofit agencies. Not all physicians will be equally responsible, nor will they be immune from responding to preferred practice styles, patient demands, or other contingencies extraneous to the clinical decision. Overall, however, this approach is preferable to the price rationing and explicit rationing alternatives.

Establishing a global budget and remunerating physicians on salary, capitation, or fees tied to an established remuneration target would weaken the current incentives for performing technical procedures that are unlikely to provide much benefit. Global budgeting will potentially provide an educational context in which, on the basis of evidence, physicians will be more open to suggestions to moderate resource utilization because they have less economic stake in performing procedures. There is also a risk of underservice, even though physicians are well socialized to be agents for patients and to balk at organizational pressures that subvert their sense of clinical responsibility (Freidson 1975).

Making physicians responsible for allocation decisions offers additional advantages. The clinician is more likely to understand the complexity of the patient's clinical condition, the social and familial consequences of the illness, patient and family preferences for conservative or aggressive care, and the value placed on possible future outcomes. Patients vary enormously in their willingness and ability to withstand pain and discomfort, to tolerate uncertainty, to fight to overcome illness, and even to stay alive. Although physicians' information on these issues is incomplete and inadequate, they have far more awareness and sensitivity than bureaucrats who typically have little or no recent clinical experience and are distant from the clinical situation. Research in psychology has shown that as decision makers become more distant, they are more likely to inflict pain (Milgram 1969). The clinical encounter remains a complex psychosocial transaction with powerful opportunities to affect the course of illness through the expectancies conveyed by the physician and the patient's development of emotional attachment and dependence (Frank and Frank 1991). Weakening this aspect of the clinical encounter by transforming the physician's function to limited technical roles would undermine important elements in the care process.

Although medical care involves numerous routine services, public concern focuses on situations of uncertainty, in which patients are seriously ill. The processes of care are sequential and iterative; both technical medical decisions and patients' personal assessments depend in part on how the processes of care unfold. Few other services involve the magnitude of personal priority and emotional involvement associated with a serious illness. Patients therefore want a physician whose judgment they trust. As Kenneth Arrow noted, if patients knew how "to measure the value of information, [they] would know the information itself. But information, in the form of skilled care, is precisely what is being bought from most physicians" (Arrow 1963:946). Patients may seek information from knowledgeable friends and other patients, medical literature, or data and advice from consumer groups, but in no way can they "test the product before consuming it" (p. 949). Thus, trust plays a key role in seeking the medical care product of any physician.

From Advocacy to Allocation

A major objection to rationing through establishing fixed budgets is that it shifts the role of physician from advocating the individual patient's needs to balancing those needs against the need to use resources responsibly so that the health care needs of the many may be met (Mechanic 1986). The claim is that such conflicting responsibilities dilute the physician's primary responsibility to "do everything in his power to alleviate [the patient's] needs" (Fried 1976). Implicit rationing, the critics argue, makes medicine subservient to two masters, undermining the ethical substructure of the physician-patient relationship.

At a theoretical level this point is unassailable if the physician's exclusive responsibility to the patient is accepted. In practice, however, limits have always existed on such advocacy, not the least of which came from the conflicting economic and social interests of the physician. The willingness of physicians to provide care and the intensity of the care provided are influenced by the patient's ability to pay and by the scope of their insurance coverage. Payment incentives, particularly fee-for-service payment, increase the provision of services. George Eliot in her classic novel *Middlemarch* noted the incentives to overprescribe among physicians who compounded their own medications. A contemporary version of this pattern is found among physicians who maintain or have equity shares in diagnostic equipment, clinical laboratories, or specialized treatment facilities to which they refer patients (Hillman et al. 1990).

The realities of practice organization also make the theoretical ethic of exclusive loyalty to the patient specious. Many physicians work for companies, insurance programs, multispecialty group practices, the government, and other organizations. As a result, these physicians accommodate competing values, colleague inclinations, organizational requirements, and the need for continued institutional viability. In many instances of serious illness, chronic disease, and long-term care, the physician's role involves the adjudication of both patient and family interests, with the doctor functioning as a negotiator and conciliator, rather than as an unfettered agent.

In fact, in the area of chronic mental illness, the National Alliance for the Mentally Ill has assailed the notion of physician as exclusive agent as a major impediment to care. It has attacked professionals who used this ethic to distance families from treatment and rehabilitation processes. Alliance members maintain that such an orientation puts the patient at risk, increases the probability of treatment failure, and imposes major costs on family and community. Psychiatrists and other mental health professionals are learning to incorporate these concerns into patient management activities, and families are increasingly involved in treatment planning.

The physician's advocacy for the patient is a value of importance, worthy of vigorous protection, but it is not absolute. Most physicians are individually responsible for at least several hundred patients and must apportion their time and efforts in some reasonable relationship to their competing patients' needs—as well as to their own needs for leisure. Some, perhaps most, patients could benefit from more time and solicitude, but the real world demands that the physician's response be appropriate, not necessarily optimal. In theory, everyone might have the same level of medical services as the president of the United States, but medical care is a process better described as "satisficing" (Simon 1957). A stronger accountability system is possible if we acknowledge and address realities rather than blindly endorse concepts that even under simple conditions of practice could be implemented only partially.

In principle, patients should understand the operating assumptions of their health program, and this is particularly critical in multichoice situations in which patients select among varying options. For many people, HMOs, and related managed care options, will offer an excellent combination of features and services providing good value for money, but it is important that they clearly understand the tradeoffs involved. Fundamentally, patients must understand that, under managed care, the role of the physician as the patient's agent and advocate may shift in subtle ways to one in which the physician consciously balances her actions on behalf of the patient against budgetary considerations.

The idea that one's physician balances interventions against cost or other considerations makes some patients uncomfortable. In a recent study of a university employment group, comprised of a majority of well-educated and sophisticated consumers, almost two-thirds of those choosing between an HMO and a traditional plan rated "feeling that your doctor is only concerned about your health and not about limiting the plan's cost" very important (Mechanic et al. 1990). Only two other considerations were more important: getting an appointment with your doctor quickly when you want one and feeling your doctor's concern about your health is his or her primary commitment. The vast majority of new HMO enrollees believed that "in this plan the doctor is only concerned about my health and not limiting the plan's cost," a perception that was in error. Despite the assumption that enrollees will learn about rationing processes quickly, the full implications of rationing are not likely to be salient until serious illness strikes and expensive diagnostic approaches, referrals, inpatient admissions, and rehabilitative technologies are at issue.

HMOs are commonly marketed with the rhetoric that they keep people healthy and contain costs by avoiding serious illness. A more accurate, but less common, representation is that HMOs offer a more comprehensive benefit package without additional out-of-pocket expenditures in exchange for the patient's acceptance of the primary physician as gatekeeper and some rationing consistent with the physician's best judgment. HMO physicians continue to view themselves primarily as their patients' agents and, probably, rarely compromise their professional judgments regarding appropriateness of care. On the margin, or in situations of uncertainty, however, the incentives of implicit rationing tilt care in a different direction than is typical in fee-for-service practice.

The HMO and managed care contract should be explicit and every potential enrollee should know to what degree their gatekeeper/physician's personal remuneration is contingent upon staying within utilization targets. Furthermore, patients have a right to know about any other financial incentives for physicians to limit expenditures and about their physician's personal economic holdings in facilities to which they are referred.

Explicit Constraints on Professional Judgment

Physicians' professional judgment should be protected, but the range of their discretion could be constrained considerably by broader political and regulatory decisions. How much to invest in medical care and the availability of technology and services are political, not medical, judgments. Public attitudes suggest that Americans will not tolerate a tightly rationed health care system that withholds efficacious, though expensive, technologies. Although Americans tend to focus on dramatic and highly expensive technologies as sources of potentially large savings, the use of such technologies is relatively infrequent. Therefore, fewer opportunities to contain costs will be realized by limiting infrequent but expensive procedures than in limiting more common procedures.

Expenditures are a product of the prevalence of interventions multiplied by unit cost. Much of the cost of medical care is an aggregation of small and intermediate cost procedures repeated frequently and among large numbers of patients, such as common radiology and laboratory procedures. Similarly, surgical procedures of moderate cost, because they are performed commonly, account for major financial outlays. Some of the most common inpatient diagnostic and surgical procedures for men are CAT scans, diagnostic ultrasound, cardiac catheterization, prostatectomy, reduction of fractures, coronary bypass, and repair of inguinal hernia (National Center for Health Statistics 1990). The most frequent female procedures are associated with reproduction, including procedures to assist delivery, cesarean sections, repair of obstetrical lacerations, and hysterectomies.

Rationing discussions often focus on relatively uncommon procedures such as heart, lung, and liver transplants. At present, these extraordinary and highly expensive procedures involve relatively few people because of the difficulty of organ procurement. Thus, expenditures on these high-cost procedures remain small and are not a serious threat to the overall health budget (Evans 1991). Advances in surgery and in the acquisition and preservation of organs could significantly increase the number of potential recipients. The experience of the Medicare End Stage Renal Disease (ESRD) Program suggests that potential growth of such programs will result from improvements in medical and surgical techniques and the availability of a financing source. This program, which covered 16,600 enrollees at an expenditure of $184 million in 1974 is estimated to have covered 93,600 enrollees in 1991 at a cost of $3.7 billion (Health Care Financing Administration 1987). As the program grows, the enrollees covered have become older and sicker and have more comorbidity and less potential for rehabilitation.

The experience of the Medicare ESRD Program has shown that the availability of an entitlement to a procedure under Medicare encourages aggressive treatment even though the benefits may be questionable. The quality of life that can be anticipated in these critical situations depends on the medical circumstances of the patients and their motivation to struggle with their condition. Age, for example, is clearly associated with the extent of comorbidity and patient condition. Yet, because of the large variance in both condition and motivation of members of any age group, age alone cannot serve as a proxy. Thus, once an entitlement to medical care becomes available, decisions about treatment must depend on careful clinical and psychosocial judgments of patient condition and motivation.

A core dilemma of such decision making is the difficulty of distinguishing clinical judgments from normative assessments and the extent to which these issues become intermingled in an implicit rationing process. Physicians commonly project their own values onto their patients in making judgments about patient motivation, capacity, function, and quality of life. Thomas Halper, for example, offers numerous examples in which physicians made unwarranted assumptions of who would or would not benefit from treatment based on judgments of intelligence, involvement in gainful employment, and worthiness (Halper 1985). Such judgments, however, are not explicit, but are deeply embedded in the processes of clinical decision making and are thus not open to discussion or review.

The dilemma faced by physicians in making implicit rationing decisions is similar to the dilemma underlying the "defensive medicine" claim in the malpractice area. Physicians commonly complain of wasteful use of expensive modalities that they deem necessary to protect themselves against allegations of malpractice. Failure to perform these procedures, however, involves a risk because other informed physicians believe these procedures to be necessary for competent treatment and will testify accordingly. The dilemma arises from the uncertainty associated with defining what constitutes a reasonable quality of care and whether nonperformance of particular tests and procedures that rarely yield new information or positive outcomes is justifiable. In rationing, as in malpractice assessment, it will be necessary to establish clearer norms defining the appropriate thresholds for additional diagnostic interventions. Everyone agrees that it makes little sense to perform a CAT scan on every patient with a headache. It is more difficult, however, to achieve a consensus on appropriate utilization boundaries.

The interconnections between social norms and medical assessments reflect the fact that doctors have social as well as technical medical functions. We expect them to become involved in the patient's world and in how the social and psychological context shapes the course of illness and treatment. Therefore, the danger is not so much that physicians consciously impose their values on patients who come from different life circumstances, but that their normative judgments are so taken for granted that they are no longer subject to circumspection. Although some inequities can be reduced by sensitizing and educating doctors about social and ethical dilemmas, by encouraging peer questioning, and by making patients more equal partners in decision making, this danger is the price of professional discretion.

Thus, initially, the threshold decision of whether to provide a new entitlement is clearly an issue with political implications and consequences. However, once the entitlement is available, the most constructive way of controlling its cost is to constrain supply and allow expert professionals to allocate treatment. This is not to say implicit rationing does not have some serious difficulties. Allocation of services through clinical judgment of patient condition and motivation requires built-in safeguards for resolving contested cases, but as a medical care rationing approach it offers the most *realistic* model for dealing with the complexities and uncertainties of clinical situations.

What Can We Learn from International Comparisons?

The most widely discussed and influential study of rationing, by Henry Aaron and William Schwartz, compared how England and the United States managed a range of technologies and treatments (Aaron and Schwartz 1984). Large differences in the uses of various treatments and technologies were reported, but the extent of rationing depended on the area of concern. Treatment for hemophilia, radiation therapy, and chemotherapy for cancer were used with comparable frequency in the two countries. Similarly, the frequency of hip replacement did not vary much, although the waiting period was longer in England. In contrast, coronary artery surgery was ten times more frequent in the United States, and dialysis and uncertain cancer treatments were less frequently utilized in England.

Interpreting these results requires some understanding of context of health care provision in each country. Aaron and Schwartz selected England, a Western nation with highly constrained investment in its health sector. At the time of the study, hospital expenditures per capita were less than half of those in the United States, largely as a result of a relatively low investment in technology. However, by selecting relatively expensive technological approaches—several of dubious value in reducing mortality or improving the quality of life—the study offers only a partial comparison. For example, England guarantees everyone access to a general practitioner, while millions in the United States face significant access barriers to primary medical care services. The United States, on the other hand, aggressively uses expensive technologies, which are more prevalent because of the incentives in fee-for-service and procedure-based reimbursement. Moreover, within Britain's health care budget, significant priority is given to the social care of the mentally ill and frail elderly persons, areas in which the U.S. health care system has major deficiencies. In contrast, the United States severely rations the availability of public services for persons with psychiatric disabilities, substance abusers, and other populations with extensive disabilities. Had Aaron and Schwartz chosen a different sample of health services, a somewhat different picture of the rationing processes might have been conveyed.

Nevertheless, Aaron and Schwartz provide a valuable analysis of the influences that result in different degrees of rationing. These influences include the age of the patient, the nature of the disease, the visibility of the disease, public advocacy, aggregate cost implications, need for capital outlays, and costs of alternatives to active care. They observe that the British disproportionately invest their health funds in children—119 percent of expenditures per adult, as compared with the United States' 37 percent. Analysts in the United States have been critical of the relatively low investment in the health care of children, attributing the situation in part to the comparative disadvantage of advocates for children relative to the elderly in making claims within our political process (Preston 1984). The high rates of voter participation and political organization among the elderly constitute a powerful political force and the U.S. health care system is thus heavily weighted in the direction of elderly care. In contrast, the British government has limited the capacity to provide dialysis to ESRD patients based on a clear relationship between age and restricted access. Although the British have no formal cutoff period by age, Aaron and Schwartz found, during the period of their study, that patients over age fifty-five were rarely seen as candidates for dialysis (Aaron and Schwartz 1984:34).

Rationing by Age

The reluctance of British general practitioners and medical specialists to refer older patients because of limited treatment capacity resulted in an implicit age criterion in health care rationing. The extent of knowledge of the current state of treatment, links to specialists in nephrology units, and judgments on who could benefit from treatment and how much treatment patients would receive varied among these nonnephrologists. Patients motivated to receive treatment, regardless of age, who were sufficiently aggressive, and who received the support of a referring physician, might receive treatment given the informality of the referral process. Referring doctors, aware of resource realities, were less likely to try to achieve referral of more frail patients, thus informally helping to adjust demand to capacity. Aaron and Schwartz reported considerable discomfort among general practitioners who were advising elderly patients with ESRD that little could be done.

The conclusions reported by Aaron and Schwartz on age rationing have commonly been exaggerated. In comparing Britain with Italy, West Germany, France, and the United States, they reported that as age increased, the disparity in rates of dialysis between Britain and these other nations increased. Data reported on renal replacement therapy in Newcastle upon Tyne, however, for the period of 1974 to 1985, suggests a growing proportion of unit patients over age sixty, due in part to changing technology and attitudes (Tapson et al. 1987). In the mid-1970s, only 2.2 percent to 7 percent of patients initiating treatment were over age sixty; by 1985, such patients starting treatment constituted more than one-third of all patients on dialysis.

Nonnephrologist discretion within the British implicit rationing approach serves a variety of functions. It allows a general practitioner or medical specialist to take into account not only chronological age, but also the health status and robustness of the individual and the potential benefits that dialysis might offer under varying circumstances. It also allows for some flexibility in responding to patient and family motivation, persistence in seeking treatment, and tensions that develop in the clinical situation.

Alternatively, the British could have used an explicit rationing approach by establishing formal criteria, which strictly rationed by age. While such a measure might have provided an illusion of equity with respect to age, it would have been difficult to administer. Moreover, the British public would have found such a clear formal mandate conceptually unacceptable. It is one matter to consider age tempered by thoughtful clinical judgment; it is quite another to impose an inflexible blanket age rule.

Daniel Callahan has suggested that we place limits "on the length of individual lives that a society can sensibly be expected to maintain" (Callahan 1986). He urges us to desist from pursuing goals that primarily benefit the elderly because they will result in increasing disparity between our aspirations and our ability to meet them. His contention that the elderly should die gracefully, without undue demand on the "medical commons," is flawed by its dependence on chronological age as an explicit criterion (Mechanic 1989). People age in varying ways, and members of any given age group are heterogeneous with respect to physical health status, psychological well-being, and ability to carry out daily living tasks. Thus, even though chronological age is a convenient administrative marker and formal age rules have the appearance of equity, large inequities become evident when circumstances other than chronological age are considered.

Many elderly persons have extraordinary capacities, extensive and intimate social ties, and a great zest for living. Unfortunately, attempts to explicitly define these capacities as criteria in any reasonable way are extremely difficult and likely to frustrate even the most expert administrative authority. Therefore, even though the use of medical criteria for assessing the value of an uncertain intervention may result in fewer interventions for the elderly, the criteria should remain the physician-determined effectiveness of the intervention and its likely benefits on a case-by-case basis.

Explaining American-British Differences

Aaron and Schwartz (1984) offer a variety of plausible hypotheses to explain why American and British practices diverge more in some areas than others, but some of these post hoc explanations are not persuasive. For example, they suggest that the similarity in cancer therapy between the two countries reflects the fear that cancer inspires in the public. Similarly, they argue that public responses to the visibility of suffering accounts for comparable responses for hemophilia relative to the large differences in the use of coronary bypass surgery.

There are numerous examples suggesting that fear of illness and visibility of suffering are inadequate or incomplete explanations for the differences in treatment approaches between the two nations. Such diseases as schizophrenia and Alzheimer's disease are fearsome and highly visible, yet they have not resulted in comparable British and American efforts to ensure the essential services needed. The British tend to be utilitarian in orientation while Americans tend to be aggressively interventionist (Payer 1988). The British have given a higher priority to noninterventionist care for the fragile elderly and the chronically mentally ill than has the American health care system. This prioritizing reflects a greater concern in British society for the caring dimensions of health interventions. The relatively low rate of coronary bypass surgery, CAT scans, and uncertain cancer interventions in England substantially reflects resource constraints, but also reflects skepticism of the true need and value of these interventions. In addition, the British response reflects widespread belief that these procedures are overutilized in the American context, often because of economic incentives.

One utilitarian approach to rationing is to extend care more widely, but to limit services to those believed to be most important or effective. In 1989, Oregon passed legislation extending Medicaid to a larger population while providing a new and more restrictive selection of benefits to a subset of Medicaid recipients. The Oregon plan divided medical services into 709 categories, but anticipated that only the first 588 would be reimbursed. Earlier drafts of this priority list were greatly criticized, partly for violating the "rule of rescue" (Hadorn 1991). The initial list of conditions rated minor treatments more highly than some life-saving measures, ostensibly reflecting cost-effectiveness considerations. For example, tooth capping was given a slightly higher priority rating than surgery for ectopic pregnancy or appendectomy, procedures that could be life-saving.

Commenting on Oregon's utilitarian approach, David Hadorn notes that "there is a fact about the human psyche that will inevitably trump the utilitarian rationality that is implicit in cost-effectiveness analysis: people cannot stand idly by when an identified person's life is visibly threatened if effective rescue measures are available" (Hadorn 1991:2218–19). Hadorn makes an important point but overstates it. It is unlikely the public will accept an explicit directive that withholds a life-saving procedure, preferring instead comparable decisions to withhold services case-by-case in clinical transactions. The British system of rationing functions with little conflict because it incorporates normative judgments as part of the process of clinical decision making. The public seems better prepared to allow such decisions to evolve in relationships between patients and their physicians.

The "rule of rescue" and the fact that such rescues involve modest aggregate costs is a more credible explanation for the full treatment of hemophilia in England than the one provided by Aaron and Schwartz. As of 1984, there were fewer than 100 new cases of hemophilia diagnosed each year in Britain, and the costs of treatment were reported to be in the $10,000–20,000 range. In contrast, the number of patients and potential aggregate costs involved in dialysis are substantially greater. As the extent of rationing of dialysis by age became more widely known—probably in part due to the publicity generated by the Aaron and Schwartz book—the British government responded by expanding dialysis capacity. The number of patients treated for ESRD in Britain increased from 153 to 242 per million population between 1983 and 1986 (Health Care Financing Administration 1989). This response indicates that the ability of the British bureaucracy to maintain constraints depends substantially on the insulation of its decisions from the political process.

The American public would not accept the constraints typical of the British system, nor can we insulate budgeting decisions from the political process as successfully as the English. Interest group pressure is likely to play a more significant role in the United States. The politics of priority setting and investments in research, technologies, and services are routinely influenced by advocacy organizations. For example, aggressive advocates have gained coverage of ESRD by Medicare, illustrating a form of selective coverage widely viewed as a poor example of how to devise health policy (Institute of Medicine 1973). A recent effort to discontinue the National Institutes of Health research program on the artificial heart was rejected by Congress in response to vigorous and influential advocates. American health care is meticulously scrutinized by a wide range of interest groups and the mass media. For example, the close scrutiny of developments in AIDS research by advocacy groups allows them to influence how the condition is defined, the manner of carrying out and regulating clinical trials, the availability and pricing of drugs, and other relevant public health policies. Similarly, the media is likely to remain vigilant, keeping close check on emerging knowledge and technology as well as on the rapidity of their application. Thus, as the American system moves toward more serious rationing, it is likely to do so under the intense scrutiny of an interested and informed public.

Making Implicit Rationing Systems Accountable

Implicit rationing is often insulated from public view and is thus susceptible to abuse. One advantage of explicit decisions is that they are visible and can be debated in the media and other forums. The public nature of explicit rationing, however, is easily exaggerated; many administrative decisions are highly technical and do not attract public attention. Powerful interest groups with high levels of technical expertise commonly negotiate compromises outside the view of other interested parties with less expertise and access to the political process. Many factors contribute to disparities in access, including the existing distribution of health facilities, the varying capacities of institutions to apply new technologies and to attract new programs and grants, the preferences and vocational decisions of health professionals, and the politics of the budgeting process itself. In sum, there is little evidence to support the idealized notion that an explicit budget process inevitably levels the playing field.

Achieving Accountability

An accountable implicit rationing system must meet three initial conditions to some extent. First, mechanisms must be in place to restrain variabilities in practice that cannot be justified by differences in the morbidity of patient populations or by clinical uncertainty. As noted throughout, while the boundaries of treatment will have to remain flexible because much remains to be learned about what is truly good practice, physician groups must, at the very least, regulate peers who transcend any reasonable or professionally justifiable basis for unusual practices. Second, physicians must agree to and support remunerative arrangements that use incentives to encourage balanced and effective care. Third, physician groups must be vigilant to ensure that services are allocated fairly, based on need and not in response to the most sophisticated, aggressive, and demanding patients. Increased sensitivity to this issue and clear norms reinforced by physician peer groups and outside review can reduce differential treatment according to socioeconomic status, race, gender, or other personal characteristics.

Deterrents to Withholding Beneficial Services

On the margins economic incentives work, although the professionalism of most physicians moderate their influence. Regardless of professionalism claims, however, implicit rationing is partly acceptable because most physicians—by training and inclination—are highly professional, resist inappropriate organizational pressures, and practice at a high ethical level (Hillman 1987). Personal remuneration arrangements that improperly modify medical decision making by providing economic incentives to doctors to withhold services should be prohibited. Comparable concerns apply to fee-for-service practitioners whose decisions to do more in marginal situations are affected by payment incentives. Patients are in a somewhat better position to refuse unwanted services or ask for second opinions in fee-for-service settings. In contrast, most patients may not even be aware of treatment possibilities when services are withheld. Therefore, deterrents to withholding services require closer scrutiny and regulation.

Although the tort system has many deficiencies, the threat of malpractice may also help deter denial of obvious beneficial services. Americans typically expect aggressive intervention, and denial of an essential service is grist for the malpractice mill. Furthermore, because standards in the United States are high, courts and juries are unlikely to be sympathetic to the denial of services known to be efficacious. Alternative mechanisms can also be developed to allow disaffected patients to appeal the refusal of a service they believe to be necessary. Such mechanisms would contribute to reducing doctor/patient tensions and would provide a window for monitoring decision making at the margins.

All systems of implicit rationing, such as HMOs, should have highly visible, accessible, and easily usable grievance mechanisms that facilitate the review of denials of service that patients believe they should receive. These mechanisms might be structured as a hierarchy of procedures ranging from the highly informal to more formal adjudication. The process might begin with an ombudsperson who negotiates disagreements between patients and their providers, with unresolved issues reviewed by an institutional committee representing the plan, clinicians, and patients. Such procedures could serve as a buffer against litigation that is slow and costly for all involved, and does not typically result in an equitable resolution of conflicts.

A major protection against underservice is careful review and periodic audits in problematic areas of care. As physicians become more aware of sharing a "medical commons," they will have a greater stake in ensuring that resources are used wisely and effectively. To the extent that physicians must consciously function within such constraints, they will be more thoughtful about aggressive care when the value of intervention is uncertain. Physicians prefer action, but functioning under implicit constraints can temper these inclinations, particularly if the action is of little or no value. One risk is that physicians as a group may adopt highly conservative norms that restrain colleagues whose best judgment leads to more interventionist practices. At present, however, American medical care is aggressively interventionist and the dangers of restraint are more theoretical than real.

Deterrents to Providing Unwanted Services

The attraction of American doctors to technology, even when there are no benefits, requires intense scrutiny. One example relates to highly technological efforts to delay the end of life. This technology incurs substantial costs when many patients and their families would prefer a less dramatic and less prolonged death. There is increasing public interest in living wills, medical powers of attorney, and related concepts, and studies suggest that a majority of persons believe they would not choose life-sustaining treatment if they had a poor prognosis (Emanuel et al. 1991). Physicians remain resistant to discussing "do-not-resuscitate" orders and related concerns with their patients, a type of interaction which they find uncomfortable. Similarly, many patients prefer less aggressive treatment alternatives than many physicians are inclined to provide. When patients are actually given options, many choose more limited approaches than physicians would have anticipated (Wennberg 1990). There is ample opportunity to involve patients to a much larger degree in choices about their own treatment. The growing interest in assisted death reflects increasing public unease with the perils of medicine's technological imperative.

One example of a highly expensive modality is intensive care, which costs approximately four times more per day than an ordinary hospital stay (Kalb and Miller 1989). If every seriously ill patient received intensive care, the aggregate costs would be extremely high. It makes little sense to use this expensive modality for patients whose prognosis is clearly hopeless or for those with little expected future quality of life. Nor is it justifiable for patients who are likely to do equally well with less intensive and expensive care.

Intelligent treatment and referral decisions depend on solid knowledge of what works and what is cost-effective. Our current knowledge is too uncertain to set specific criteria for admission and discharge, but research on outcomes may inform decisions about the value of alternative interventions. Even the most sophisticated clinical trials, however, are limited to select groups of patients who meet study criteria and may not represent the populations that physicians may typically see. Thus, even when rigorous research results are available, determining their applicability to patients with different social and clinical characteristics involves extrapolation. Over time, models, based on refined medical criteria, are likely to develop. Because of variation in the circumstances of patients, these models cannot be mechanically applied, but they can provide guidance for physicians to consider as they struggle with clinical decisions under uncertainty.

Tragic Choices

The allocation of scarce resources, as in the case of organ transplantation, is not prototypical of the majority of rationing decisions made within our vast health care system. Decisions about the allocation of scarce life-saving resources, however, will become more common with technological advances and will receive a great deal of publicity. These decisions detract attention from the far more numerous circumstances under which more routine types of rationing occur.

The problem with the dramatic case of who gets the heart and lung transplant among equally medically eligible recipients is that there is no answer, and resolution requires an arbitrary decision among competing values. To the extent that predictive medical models can be improved it may be possible to make finer biological gradations in ranking those most likely to benefit. The discriminations, however, may become so small as to have little practical import. Maintaining the illusion that only medical criteria are operative makes it possible to avoid agonizing choices among competing values.

An alternative, of course, in deciding among equally medically eligible recipients is simply to distribute available shares by lottery. Although a lottery offers the only fair resolution among conflicting values, it encounters great resistance from the public and professionals who prefer criteria of worthiness for these extraordinarily expensive decisions. If we choose to discriminate among recipients on some worthiness criteria, it is imperative that this be done by a fair and legitimate process that incorporates a wide range of competing viewpoints.

Conclusion

Societies will expend enormous resources to rescue persons trapped in a mine, lost at sea, and on many other accidental occasions. Such rescues are symbolic, affirming the value of life and the commitment of the community to individuals in distress. It seems likely that if such accidents occurred more routinely, the intensity of these rescue efforts would diminish. Similarly, many new medical techniques begin as rescues and have major symbolic as well as research significance, but as these dramatic rescue efforts become viable for larger populations of patients they raise imposing allocation questions. A heart-lung transplant may cost well over a hundred thousand dollars initially with subsequent yearly costs of approximately $50,000. Our capacity to carry out very few rescues has little impact on the health care system as a whole, but if many thousands were possible the situation would change.

Rescues eventually become viable as "conventional care," and great pressures develop to insure for them. Had policymakers realized the cost of covering ESRD under Medicare they would have entered this arena more carefully. It was inevitable that dialysis coverage would have been extended because in the American context, with its emphasis on the worth of the individual, the notion of rescue carries great weight. Once the capability is acquired, there is extensive public pressure to use it if life is at stake. Given this reality, some have suggested that we should focus our research and development investments on cost-effective technologies and on those that are cost saving. It remains unclear that this would be politically viable given public attitudes and the pressures from the various constituencies that have a major stake in current research and technological developments.

The question of how long American society can delay coming to terms with the rationing issue in an open manner remains unanswered. Each year, as costs mount and new possibilities accelerate, the notion that we can muddle along in the usual way becomes less tenable. Even if such strategies as those represented in the Oregon Plan were feasible on a broad scale, a conclusion undermined by the exclusions negotiated in Oregon's political process (Brown 1991), it is not clear that the decisions can be implemented successfully in a manner that makes sense clinically. Helping is a holistic process, not easily divided into artificial categories of care. Medicine cannot ignore caring without destroying much of the value and significance of the therapeutic encounter. Given these realities, it seems most reasonable for society to set whatever constraints on medical care expenditures that are politically necessary and leave microdecisions to negotiations between patients and health professionals. These decisions, however, should be carried out in a context of universal health care in which the entire population has access to a basic, decent, minimal standard of care.

References

Aaron, H.J. and Schwartz, W.B. 1984. *The Painful Prescription: Rationing Hospital Care.* Washington, DC: The Brookings Institution.
Arrow, K.J. 1963. "Uncertainty and the welfare economics of medical care." *American Economic Review* 53:941–49.
Brown, L.D. 1991. "The national politics of Oregon's rationing plan." *Health Affairs* 10:28–51.

Calabresi, G. 1974. "Commentary." In Trancredi, L.R. (ed.), *Ethics of Health Care.* Washington, DC: Institute of Medicine, National Academy of Sciences, 48–55.

Callahan, D. 1986. "Adequate health care and an aging society: Are they morally compatible?" *Daedalus* 115:247–67.

Chassin, M.R., Kosecoff, J., Park, R.E., Winslow, C.M., Kahn, K.L., Merrick, N.J., Keesey, J., Fink, A., Solomon, D.H., and Brook, R.H. 1987. "Does inappropriate use explain geographic variations in the use of health care services: A study of three procedures." *Journal of the American Medical Association* 258:2533–37.

Eddy, D.M. 1984. "Variations in physician practice: The role of uncertainty." *Health Affairs* 3:74–90.

Emanuel, L.L., Barry, M.J., Stoeckle, J.D., Ettelson, L.M., and Ezekiel, J.E. 1991. "Advance directives for medical care: A case for greater use." *New England Journal of Medicine* 324:889–95.

Enthoven, A. 1985. "Health tax policy mismatch." *Health Affairs* 4:5–14.

Evans, R.W. 1991. "Organ transplantation costs, insurance coverage, and reimbursement." In Terasaki, P.I. (ed.), *Clinical Transplants 1990.* Los Angeles, CA: UCLA Tissue Typing Laboratories, 319–25.

Frank, J.D., and Frank, J.B. 1991. *Persuasion and Healing,* 3rd ed. Baltimore: Johns Hopkins University Press.

Freidson, E. 1975. *Doctoring Together: A Study of Professional Social Control.* New York: Elsevier.

Fried, C. 1976. "Equality and rights in medical care." *Hastings Center Report* 34:29–34.

Friedman, L.M. 1971. "The idea of right as a social and legal concept." *Journal of Social Issues* 27:189–98.

Hadorn, DC 1991. "Setting health care priorities in Oregon: Cost-effectiveness meets the rule of rescue." *Journal of the American Medical Association* 265:2218–25.

Halper, T. 1985. "Life and death in a welfare state: End-stage renal disease in the United Kingdom," *The Milbank Quarterly* 63:52–93.

Health Care Financing Administration. 1989. *Health Care Financing Review, Annual Supplement.* Baltimore, MD: U.S. Dept. of Health and Human Services, p. 174, table 47.

———. 1987. *Health Care Financing Special Report: Findings from the National Kidney Dialysis and Kidney Transplantation Study.* Baltimore MD: U.S. Dept. of Health and Human Services, 26–27.

Hillman, A.L. 1987. "Financial incentives for physicians in HMOs: Is there a conflict of interest?" *New England Journal of Medicine* 317:1743–48.

Hillman, B.J., Joseph, C.A., Mabry, M.R., Sunshine, J.H., Kennedy, S.D., and Noether, M. 1990. "Frequency and costs of diagnostic imaging in office practice: A comparison of self-referring and radiologist-referring physicians." *New England Journal of Medicine* 323:1604–08.

Institute of Medicine. 1973. *Disease by Disease: Toward National Health Insurance?—Report of a Panel: Implications of a Categorical Catastrophic Disease Approach to National Health Insurance.* Washington, DC: National Academy Press.

Kalb, P.E., and Miller, D.H. 1989. "Utilization strategies for intensive care units." *Journal of the American Medical Association* 261:2389-95.

Knaus, W.A., Wagner, D.P., and Lynn, J. 1991. "Short-term mortality predictions for critically ill hospitalized adults: Science and ethics." *Science* 254:389-94.

Lazenby, H.C., and Letsch, S.W. 1989. "National health expenditures 1989." *Health Care Financing Review* 12:1-26.

Leape, L.L., Park, R.E., Solomon, D.H., Chassin, M.R., Kosecoff, J., and Brook, R.H. 1990. "Does inappropriate use explain small-area variations in the use of health care services." *Journal of the American Medical Association* 263:669-72.

Lohr, K.N., Brook, R.H., Kamberg, C.J., Goldberg, G.A., Leibowitz, A., Keesey, Jr., Reboussin, D., and Newhouse, J.P. 1986. *Use of Medical Care in the Rand Health Insurance Experiment: Diagnosis- and Service-Specific Analyses in a Randomized Controlled Trial.* Santa Monica, CA: RAND Corporation, R-3469-HHS.

Mechanic, D. 1989. "Health care and the elderly." In Riley, M., and Riley, J. (eds.),*The Quality of Aging: Potentials for Change. Annals American Academy of Political & Social Science* 503:89-98.

_____. 1986. *From Advocacy to Allocation: The Evolving American Health Care System.* New York: Free Press.

_____. 1979. *Future Issues in Health Care: Social Policy and the Rationing of Medical Services.* New York: Free Press.

_____. 1978. *Medical Sociology,* 2d ed. New York: Free Press.

Mechanic, D., Ettel, T., and Davis, D. 1990. "Choosing among health insurance options: A study of new employees." *Inquiry* 27:14-23.

Milgram, S. 1969. *Obedience to Authority.* London: Tavistock.

National Center for Health Statistics. 1990. *Health, United States.* Pub. No. (PHS) 91-1232. Hyattsville, MD: Public Health Service.

Newhouse, J.P., Manning, W.G., Morris, C.N., Orr, L.L., Duan, N., Keeler, E.B., Leibowitz, A., Marquis, K.H., Marquis, M.S., Phelps, C.E., and Brook, R.H. 1981. "Some interim results from a controlled trial of cost sharing in health insurance." *New England Journal of Medicine* 305:1501-07.

Payer, L. 1988. *Medicine and Culture, Varieties of Treatment in the United States, England, West Germany and France.* New York: Henry Holt.

Preston, S.H. 1984. "Children and the elderly: Divergent paths for America's dependents." *Demography* 21:435-57.

Siu, A.L., Sonnenberg, F.A., Manning, W.G., Goldberg, G.A., Bloomfield, E.S., Newhouse, J.P., and Brook, R. 1986. "Inappropriate use of hospitals in a randomized trial of health insurance plans." *New England Journal of Medicine* 315:1259-66.

Simon, H.A. 1957. *Administrative Behavior.* New York: Free Press.
Tapson, J.S., Rodger, R.S.C., Mansy, H., Elliott, R.W., Ward, M.K., and Wilkinson, R. 1987. "Renal replacement therapy in patients aged over 60 years." *Postgraduate Medical Journal* 63:1071-77.
Wennberg, J.E. 1990. "Outcomes research, cost containment, and the fear of health care rationing." *New England Journal of Medicine* 323:1202-04.
White, K.L. 1988. Foreword. In Payer, L., *Medicine and Culture, Varieties of Treatment in the United States, England, Germany and France.* New York: Henry Holt, 9-10.

PART II

Need for a New Paradigm

4

Conceptions of Health

The diagnosis of disease is a highly focused activity that abstracts from what Verbrugge and Ascione (1987) have called the iceberg of symptoms, most hidden from the formal medical care system. Epidemiological studies demonstrate, in contrast, that most people have symptoms most of the time but normalize or deny them. Indeed, acute symptoms are so ubiquitous that they are impossible to measure reliably and, thus, statistical agencies will usually only count such symptoms if the respondent actually took some action in response such as self-medication or bed rest (Mechanic and Newton 1965).

In one of the classic papers in the health services field, White, Williams, and Greenberg (1961) calculated monthly prevalence and help-seeking rates from morbidity surveys in the United States and the United Kingdom. They estimated that in any given month three quarters of the population had one or more illnesses or injuries sufficiently salient to take some action. Only one in four in the population in any month sought physician care, and not all these were necessarily symptomatic. Moreover, studies of patients' presenting complaints show great overlap with untreated symptoms in the general population. Once these facts are clear, it becomes essential to inquire why patients have chosen to present their symptoms to the medical care system at the time they do, and what differentiates them from people with comparable symptoms who do not seek assistance (Balint 1957). Asking such questions about how people select themselves from a population at risk into care constitutes one aspect of the study of illness behavior, the processes involved in recognizing, defining, and making attributions about illness and what to do about it (Mechanic 1986a).

Doctors of first contact see many of the same problems commonly occurring in the population, and as Kerr White observed some years ago, almost half of the patients seen at first contact may have such vague and ambiguous presentations that they cannot be given a diagnosis that fits categories covered by the International Classification of Disease (White 1970). A substantial proportion of these patients are also depressed, anxious, and fatigued, although estimates vary wildly contingent on definition and on how such assessments are made. While there are disagreements on the precise figures, there is no disagreement that most medical problems occur in a social context complicated by issues of class, race, gender, work, family, and community ties.

Physicians throughout the world are taught to approach patients through a diagnostic process in which they elicit the chief complaint, the characteristics of the present illness, past history, and family and socially relevant factors. They then are taught to do a systems review, physical examination, and other necessary investigations leading to a diagnosis (Waitzkin 1991:25–31). They pursue this process selectively, searching for a pattern that fits preconceived disease theories. Jerome Kassirer (1992), editor of the *New England Journal of Medicine*, put it this way: "In many ways the diagnostic process resembles the start of a chess game: after one or two moves (one or two symptoms), the number of possible moves (diagnostic possibilities) is usually enormous; in both chess and medicine, the object is to win, but the challenge is to make the right move in the right direction at the right time. Unfortunately, the route is almost never clear in advance. Deciding about the use of tests or therapeutic approaches requires unstructured problem-solving because the physician is often working at the fuzzy boundaries of medical knowledge" (p. 60).

At any point in time, the practice of medicine is a mixture of theories at varying levels of confirmation and a variety of social judgments and prejudices (Mechanic 1978). Physicians seek to identify patterns of symptoms that imply definable disorder, and if they do so successfully, and the disease theory is relatively firm, they gain abundant information on likely course and etiology and guidance for how to proceed in treatment. Physician roles substantially transcend the corpus of medical knowledge, and both patients and the societies of which they are part demand that doctors provide assistance even when knowledge is limited.

Much disease and its course are influenced by social and environmental factors, but medical practice tends to personalize such influences by focusing on their individual manifestations and consequences typically divorced from broader implications. Why this particular emphasis evolved historically may seem natural to us, but it was neither self-evident nor inevitable, and it is even arguable that the approach is particularly well-fitted to much of the morbidity that doctors now treat. As Waitzkin notes,

That this particular format should have arisen is remarkable partly because its effectiveness in improving medical conditions remains unproven. Like many other aspects of modern medicine the beneficial impact of the format on the morbidity and mortality of large populations, as well as on individual patients, is difficult or impossible to demonstrate. . . . Many of the medical encounter's most time-consuming and thus costly components . . . have never been put to the test of cost-effectiveness . . . . Why has the medical encounter's traditional format received such wide and unquestioning acceptance that it is now essentially a sacred cow? (Waitzkin 1991:33)

Waitzkin, in a contextual analysis of a sample of doctor-patient contacts, observed the numerous ways in which doctors, explicitly or inadvertently, exercised social controls as they acted on traditional ideologies relating to family, work, appropriate behavior, age expectations, and the like. As he notes,

through messages of ideology and social control, and through the lack of contextual criticism, health professionals subtly direct patients' actions to conform with society's dominant expectations about appropriate behavior. . . . Doctor-patient encounters become micropolitical situations that reflect and support broader social relations, including social class and political-economic power. The participants in these encounters seldom recognize their micropolitical situation on a conscious level." (Pp. 8–9)

In the primary medical care literature, much attention is focused on the idea of the patient's hidden agenda—the "real" reason for the consultation that becomes apparent late in the transaction, if at all (Balint 1957). An alternative to the traditional approach is to give patients greater latitude to tell their stories and to explain what they expect and hope for from the encounter. As Waitzkin notes, "Most practitioners would acknowledge that the tendencies to interrupt, cut off, or otherwise redirect the patient's story during the PI [evaluation of present illness] derive at least partly from the drive to make a diagnosis. That is, a doctor wants to hear those words that are consistent with previously defined diagnostic categories. Parts of patients' stories that do not fit neatly into these categories function as unwanted strangers in medical discourse" (p. 32).

A powerful analogy comes from anthropological work on comparative law. In our legal system, courts work with an elaborate body of statutes and legal precedents that guide dispute settlements. In cases before the court, the judge's responsibility is to make decisions through the application of preexisting rules and their elaboration through application to specific cases. The judge's role is to insure that the presentation of the case follows the rules of evidence and that the issues at stake be resolved on legal principles and not on the underlying motives of the parties to the dispute or the social consequences for the litigants and their kinship group. Yet, we also know that in many instances—medical malpractice and divorce being excellent examples—the issues being litigated are often quite different from the primary dispute that brought the parties into court and not reflective of the real disagreements between them. The legal battle becomes the turf on which the real underlying dispute is played out, often in a way that further polarizes the parties, making future reconciliation impossible. Judges may be fully aware of this, but searching out the underlying problems once the issue is before the court is not really their business.

Consider, in contrast, the judicial process among the Barotse, a Northern Rhodesian tribe studied by Max Gluckman (1965). The Barotse judge explores in depth the nature of disputes seeking to resolve basic conflicts and disagreements that might extend well beyond the manifest issue. This requires far-reaching inquiry, allowing each disputant to tell his or her story in full, and encouraging the participation of other interested parties in these deliberations. Gluckman maintained that the aim of the judge, particularly in kinship disputes, was to keep kin together and maintain village integrity. The judge, thus, sees the main role as reconciling the parties and reaching a satisfactory compromise judgment.

As patterns of disease have changed, and as medicine is more concerned with chronic and degenerative diseases and behavior patterns associated with morbidity, it is appropriate to re-examine optimal approaches to identifying the real problem and alternative management strategies. Such an approach, unlike the dominant medical model, makes values and moral issues more salient. The fact that they are at present implicit in most situations makes them no less important. It may well be that an approach to the patient along the lines of the Barotse judge may be more helpful in getting to the core of essential issues.

In many encounters a negotiation process goes on in which doctor and patient agree to focus on one or another aspect of the problem in a way that may help bring the problem into congruence with an intelligible medical definition. But things are not always easy, and despite concerted efforts to identify a meaningful problem formulation, the doctor may fail to arrive at any hypothesis that fits. Physicians get frustrated with persistent and demanding patients who pose such ambiguities and label them as neurotic, "worried wells," "hypochondriacs," or "crocks." The failure to locate a suitable hypothesis may tell us as much about the physician's models and approaches as it does about the illness behavior of the patient, but the failure is usually externalized and in an invidious way. When confirmed medical models don't fit, one gets a heavy dose of social judgment often disguised as diagnosis. The characteristic inter-mixture of clinical observations with judgmental ones makes it almost impossible to separate social from technical clinical norms.

Alternative Paradigms to the Dominant Medical Model

The dominant concept of disease and the medical process of diagnostic inquiry focused on the individual, in contrast to broader systems is not inevitable or necessarily the most efficient or effective way of promoting individual health. Diagnosticians of first contact exist in every culture because people seek a place to bring difficult problems for which they seek relief, hope, and reassurance. But the point of clinical intervention is a peculiar vantage point for viewing the production of health and disease.

At the level of populations, the notion is now commonplace that health is shaped by the material and environmental conditions of life and by the sociocultural structures that people create as much as by their genes and individual health behavior. Much of positive or damaging health-relevant behaviors arise from the routine activities and conventional patterns of everyday life, only modestly influenced by health-relevant considera-tions (Mechanic 1990). The flow of health outcomes from routine processes is pervasive and powerful. The instruments to promote health, thus, are quite varied, including tax policies and other financial incen-tives, regulation, skillful use of mass media, and education. Possibilities include social policies regulating environmental and workplace risk exposures; distribution, labeling, and regulation of food, drugs, and other commodities; controls over smoking, drinking, and other high-risk behaviors; highway construction and road and vehicle safety systems; and inducements for exercise, community participation, and social integration. Focus on the personal level reflects in part the individualistic bias of Western culture. As concern with promoting health has grown, the emphasis has overwhelmingly been on personal health habits in contrast to other levels of intervention. In considering policy options, there are at least four major possible trade-offs: between macro nonhealth interventions that promote health (education, community empowerment and mobilization, social integration, inducing personal efficacy) and more direct health initiatives; between public health efforts and general medical care; between individual preventive versus curative foci; and between primary care and more specialized types of interventions. Most resource investment in the U.S. system is inversely related to the spheres of action most likely to have the largest impact on population health.

The Idea of Health

Our thinking is enriched by the perspectives of René Dubos, a microbiologist and discoverer of the source of the first commercially produced antibiotics. Dubos, seeking an enzyme to decompose the envelope protecting bacteria causing lobar pneumonia, turned his attention to the study of swamp soil where he began developing his appreciation for the richness of natural variability and its effects on the development of organisms. As he pursued his studies, Dubos became convinced that the "prevalence and severity of microbial diseases are conditioned more by the ways of life of the persons afflicted than by the virulence and other properties of the etiological agents" (Dubos 1965).

As Dubos engaged the study of disease and environment and the extraordinary adaptiveness of organisms to changing conditions, he became critical of exaggerated claims about the effectiveness of solving health problems solely through medicine. While himself an eminent medical scientist, he understood that health cannot be an absolute or permanent value, however careful the social and medical planning. As he eloquently explained, "Biological success in all its manifestations is a measure of fitness, and fitness requires never-ending efforts of adaptation to the total environment which is ever changing" (Dubos 1959).

There have been numerous efforts to define health both in general and psychological terms. Marie Jahoda (1958), for example, identified six primary themes recurring in definitions of positive mental health, such as positive attitudes toward the self, integration of personality, autonomy, and environmental mastery. The difficulty is the lack of specificity in these criteria and their dependence on social values and social judgments that may vary widely by culture and social context. As she herself noted, "there is hardly a term in current psychological thought as vague, elusive and ambiguous as the term 'mental health'" (Jahoda 1958). Yet the effort to study health as a global concept, whatever its difficulties and ambiguities, is not a fool's mission.

1. A number of important disease risk factors appear to have nonspecific effects on a wide range of disease conditions and mortality; these include broad factors such as socioeconomic status, social networks and supports, and stressful life events, as well as more specific patterns of behavior such as smoking, exercise, and intimate relations (Mechanic 1982a; Syme 1986). It is conceivable that as we learn more we will be able to account for most of these influences through specific processes linked to each disease, but the nonspecific effects are robust. Moreover, the more we learn about biological processes, the more evident it becomes that while models of specific disease syndromes are pragmatic and essential for advancements, the syndromes are related and not discrete.

2. Self-reports of health status and subjective health assessments are among the best general predictors of mortality, morbidity, and use of medical care services (Ware 1986). Various studies have found that such subjective assessments are not only significantly related to objective indicators such as physician assessments, medical record data, and mortality (LaRue et al. 1979; Ferraro 1980; Eisen et al. 1980; Fillenbaum 1979), but are independent predictors of mortality controlling for objective assessments of health and known risk factors (Mossey and Shapiro 1982; Kaplan and Camacho 1983). Mossey and Shapiro (1982), in studying 3,128 noninstitutionalized elderly people, found a threefold difference in mortality over six years between those rating their health excellent and those rating it poor, which persisted when controlled for age, sex, residence, and health status indicators. Similarly, Kaplan and Camacho (1983), in a nine-year follow-up of a large California adult sample, found large differences in mortality associated with prior sub-

jective assessments. These effects persist when controlled for baseline measures of health practices, social networks, health indicators, and psychological status. The superiority of such self-assessments over objective medical assessments is an intriguing puzzle. Idler (1992) reviewed six follow-up studies based on large probability samples that included baseline health self-assessments and objective health status measures allowing appropriate statistical analyses. These studies consistently show the influence of self-assessed health despite controls for objective health status measures.

3. There is good statistical evidence that persons can "will" their survival or death over short time spans, and that for these limited time intervals social events can be powerful predictors (Phillips and Feldman 1973; Phillips and King 1988). Moreover, relatively modest social interventions among elderly institutionalized populations show effects not only on well-being but even mortality. Langner and Rodin (1976) assessed an intervention that gave nursing home residents more choices in their everyday lives. Follow-up after eighteen months found that those in the intervention group experienced improved health as well as a marginal improvement in longevity relative to the comparison group (Rodin and Langner 1977; Rodin 1986).

4. There is substantial literature linking morbidity and mortality to patterns of industrialization, urbanization, migration, and acculturation (Dubos 1959, 1965; Grob 1983). Other powerful influences include schooling, patterns of marriage and divorce, religious and group affiliation, and community participation and employment patterns (Mechanic 1978, 1982a, 1988). Many of these data are either cross-sectional or aggregated in ways that make it impossible to differentiate cause and effect. But the literature in its totality is persuasive of the importance of depicting the role of broad processes by which the measured end results occur, and of the crucial intervening variables.

The challenge to the investigator is to dissect these enormously complicated patterns in ways that retain the meaningfulness of the original observations but with rigorous research procedures and measurement that allow testing alternative explanations.

The predictive value of simple health perceptions is remarkable, but their meaning remains uncertain. A number of studies indicate that individuals in making assessments of health adopt a holistic frame of reference that is influenced by appraisals of their ability to function and the extent to which health decrements interfere (Mechanic 1978). Even when efforts are made to focus the individual's attention on the physical dimension of health, the rating reflects broader aspects of social function and not only measurable medical morbidity or lack of physical fitness. Furthermore, such assessments seem to be made typically in terms of some standard of comparison the respondent has in mind. For example, many studies have found that elderly respondents report more positive health assessments relative to objective indicators than younger adults (Maddox and Douglass 1973; Linn and Linn 1980; Friedsam and Martin 1963; Cockerham, Sharp, and Wilcox 1983). A number of researchers have suggested that elderly persons are health optimists, but this characterization simply renames rather than illuminates the issue. One possibility is that the elderly adjust their perceptions because of health expectations that have changed as they get older (Tornstam 1975). A negative consequence of such altered expectations is that individuals may neglect remediable problems because they associate such deficits with aging rather than with disease.

In one analysis, Richard Tessler and I (Tessler and Mechanic 1978) examined four diverse data sets to ascertain the relationship between various independent predictors and persons' perceptions of their own health. Included were samples of persons participating in alternative health insurance plans, a large sample of students at a major state university, a sample of men in a state prison, and a sample of persons aged forty-five to sixty-nine in a southern state. In this analysis we were concerned with factors predicting perceived health status, controlling for measures of actual health status. The need to have a measure of objective health status, as well as some other variables, directed the choice of data sets. The particular measures used for the analysis in each of the data sets are generally comparable, although they vary somewhat. It was our view, however, that the diversity of samples and variations in measures employed were an advantage in that if the same results emerge across data sets in spite of differences, we can have increased confidence in the generality of the basis processes under study.

In each data set the dependent variable is the respondent's assessment of his or her health status, and the independent predictors consist of (1) a measure of physical health status (in two data sets we had physician ratings, while in the other two we depended on reported measures of illness); (2) a measure of psychological distress; and (3) measures of age, marital status, sex, education, and race whenever they were applicable. The main concern of the analysis was to assess the degree to which psychological distress influenced people's perceptions of their health, taking into account both sociodemographic factors and some measure of "objective physical health."

For each data set we constructed a multiple regression equation in which perceived health status was regressed simultaneously against the other variables. Psychological distress was the only variable other than the measure of physical health status that retained a statistically significant standardized beta coefficient in all four data sets. As we expected, physical health status had a larger influence on perceived health than psychological distress, although this was not true in the case of the prison sample, and the betas in the sample of older people for the two predictors were fairly close. It is worthy of note, however, that the measures of physical health status made by physicians were less powerful than those based on respondent reports of illness, suggesting that the latter are influenced by a certain degree of respondent subjectivity. This finding supported our basic contention that subjective reports of illness already reflect to some extent the psychological state of the person providing the data (Mechanic 1979).

I view the self-assessment of health as an active process involving cognitive and emotional strategies typically used in assessing the self. Thus, physical symptoms are only one of the many building blocks in forming this conception. Particular symptoms may be given prominence or may be defined as peripheral to the person's judgments of self and health. The fact that young people have little serious morbidity (Haggerty 1983) provided an opportunity to examine the constituents of health appraisals in a sample of 1,193 adolescents using longitudinal data (Mechanic and Hansell 1987). If serious illness is not a major constituent of the self-appraisal, how then do young people with little chronic disease or serious morbidity form a self-appraisal of their health? In this instance we predicted that psychological well-being and competence in age relevant areas would shape such self-conceptions.

We indeed found that adolescents who reported higher levels of school achievement and more participation in sports and other exercise assessed their health as better over a one-year period than those reporting lower achievement and less participation, controlling for self-assessed health at the beginning of the year. Other longitudinal results showed that adolescents who were initially less depressed assessed their health more positively. Our measure of common physical symptoms was associated cross-sectionally with self-assessed health, but its longitudinal effect was mediated by initial levels of self-assessed health. In short, for these adolescents health is truly a social concept that reflects psychological well-being and competence in age-appropriate activities. If we form conceptions about ourselves by observing our own behavior as Bem (1972) has suggested, then adolescents may conclude they are healthy in part because they are active and competent. Having only limited physiological feedback, they may depend on judgments of their competence and activity to appraise themselves.

If health appraisals develop in this way it becomes easier to understand why patients' presentations to physicians intermix physical symptoms, psychological distress, and psychosocial difficulties. Physicians are trained to apply a disease model that seeks discrete infirmities but patients do not typically respond to their health problems in accord with medical models. Understanding the source of these discordant definitions and how patients' conceptions are formed provides new opportunities for medical care interventions.

Illness Behavior

The study of illness behavior seeks to identify the sociocultural, psychological, and situational determinants that make people aware of symptoms, the cognitive schemata they use to interpret them, and the ways the organization and financing of services facilitate or impede varying kinds of care-seeking. Illness behavior helps shape the formation and course of illness. Illness often serves a variety of social and personal objectives that have little to do with biological systems or the pathogenesis of disease. The boundaries of illness and its definitions are extraordinarily broad, and the illness process can be used to negotiate a range of cultural, social, and personal tensions. Illness behavior is one of many alternatives for coping with personal and social tensions and conflict.

There is now an extensive literature on illness behavior (Mechanic 1978, 1982b, 1983; Kleinman 1986, 1988; McHugh and Vallis 1985), and sufficient familiarity with the concept to reduce a need for general elaboration. Here I focus on just a few points continuous with the preceding discussion on health status assessment. While we take knowing about how our body feels as self-evident, such judgments are difficult because of the absence of objective guides to which we can compare our internal experiences. Because of the absence of standards, people look to their environment or popular theories for a reasonable accounting of their experiences (Leventhal 1985). People generally believe that stress elevates blood pressure, for example, and thus, hypertensives commonly believe that their blood pressure is high when they are under stress and adapt their medications accordingly. Expecting a relation between medication and symptom change, patients typically reduce prescribed medication as symptoms abate. Medication adherence requires overcoming commonly understood popular models of cause and effect.

Very popular theories are so widely shared that both patient and doctor understand the premises upon which judgments are being made. But in many instances there are no commonly accepted conceptions, or the illness models people use are influenced by subcultures or are idiosyncratic. Thus practitioners must explore the attributions and theories that help guide the patient's responses.

Illness behavior plays an intriguing role in pain response and disability, particularly in respect to back pain (Osterweis, Kleinman, and Mechanic 1987). Spitzer and Task Force (1986), in a Canadian study, found that less than 8 percent of patients complaining of back pain not supported by objective findings became chronic. We have no adequate models that can predict which of these patients will have self-limited conditions and who will become chronic. Illness behavior plays an important role, contributing to work absenteeism, use of medical services, and demands on the disability insurance system, but the precise factors, and how they influence outcomes, are difficult to specify.

There are a number of studies demonstrating that when depression occurs concurrently with acute disease, patients may attribute to the acute disease symptoms associated with persistent depressed affect, thus prolonging the illness process (Imboden et al. 1959; Imboden et al. 1961). Such studies alert us to the fact that many patients may have difficulty interpreting the origin of symptoms when illnesses occur concomitantly. While much of the existing literature is based on the assumption that chronicity is in some sense motivated by secondary gain, the opportunities for confusion in symptom appraisal exist independently of the uses of illness to achieve advantages not otherwise available.

In a study of back pain, we had an opportunity to analyze data from the United States Health and Nutrition Examination Survey (HANES) among a subsample of 2,431 respondents for whom we had both self-report data and findings from an extensive medical examination (Mechanic and Angel 1987). This allowed development of an index that depicted the extent to which reported back pain exceeded physical findings. As in other studies, we found that older patients and those reporting higher levels of psychological well-being were less likely to make invalidated complaints, controlling for age, sex, race, marital status, education, and income. Depressed mood was associated with both more complaints and more physical findings, suggesting that causal factors operated in both directions. Our most interesting finding was that the inclination of older persons to report less pain at comparable levels of physical status based on the examination was significant only among those with higher levels of psychological well-being. This supports the notion that subjective assessments of health are made in the context of comparing oneself to others. As people age, they may attribute some of their discomforts to the aging process and, thus, are more likely to normalize bodily discomforts. Persons who, in general, are experiencing a sense of well-being may feel they are doing well relative to their reference groups. Those with depressed mood are less likely to feel so.

The tendency of patients to view their health holistically, and not in terms of discrete categories, also complicates the way they seek help and express their complaints. The association between psychological and physical symptoms is widely recognized (Eastwood 1975), and psychiatric patients are large consumers of nonpsychiatric health services (Jones and Vischi 1979) relative to the population. In a study comparing a sample of psychiatric outpatients with a representative sample from the same population from which they came (Mechanic, Cleary, and Greenley 1982), we found that the psychiatric patients made 100 percent more nonpsychiatric medical care visits in the year prior to the study and 83 percent more in the year following than those in the representative sample.

There are a variety of possible explanations. One is that the excess visit rate is largely due to physical symptoms and dysfunction concomitant with psychiatric disorder. A second is that a higher propensity to seek help contributes to both becoming a psychiatric patient and to using general medical services. A third possibility is that once a person enters the psychiatric system, access to other services is easier. We developed measures that allowed us to compare the strength of these alternative explanations. Among them, the hypothesis dealing with concomitant symptoms explained the most variance, but illness behavior propensities were also important. These results suggest that patients are often unclear about the origins of their symptoms, or the appropriate attributions and help-seeking behavior. Nor are physicians always helpful in clarifying such issues.

Conclusion

The sources of health and disease in societies are broad and complex. Communities will have different rates and patterns of pathology, depending on demographic, economic, and psychosocial influences that interact with the biological potentials and limitations of people (Mechanic 1986b, 1986c), and these patterns will be altered by changes in environmental ecology and social organization. The medical model offers a useful but limited perspective on the factors that affect the occurrence and course of disease and alternatives for prevention and control. The current AIDS crisis vividly reminds us of the influence of social organization and behavior on the transmission of disease and the role of social groupings and subcultures in its spread or control. From this perspective, the idea of health, and its broad conceptualization is hardly unimportant. Definition and measurement are central to the challenge but to allow the easily measurable to guide our definitions of what is important and our research efforts would be exceedingly foolish.

References

Bem, D. 1972. "Self-perception theory." In Berkowitz, L. (ed.), *Advances in Experimental Social Psychology 6*. New York: Academic Press, 2–62.
Balint, M. 1957. *The Doctor, His Patient and the Illness*. New York: International Universities Press.
Cockerham, W.C., Sharp, K., and Wilcox, J.A. 1983. "Aging and perceived health status." *Journal of Gerontology* 38:349–55.
Dubos, R. 1965. *Man Adapting*. New Haven: Yale University Press.
_____. 1959. *Mirage of Health: Utopias, Progress, and Biological Change*. New York: Harper.
Eastwood, M.R. 1975. *The Relation Between Physical and Mental Illness*. Toronto: University of Toronto Press.

Eisen, M., Donald, C.A., Ware, J.E. Jr., and Brook, R.H. 1980. *Conceptualization and Measurement of Health for Children in the Health Insurance Study.* R-2312-HEW. Santa Monica, CA: Rand Corporation.

Ferraro, K.F. 1980. "Self-ratings of health among the old and the old-old." *Journal of Health and Social Behavior* 21:377-83.

Fillenbaum, G.G. 1979. "Social context and self-assessment of health among the elderly." *Journal of Health and Social Behavior* 20:45-51.

Friedsam, H., and Martin, H.W. 1963. "A comparison of self and physicians' ratings in an older population." *Journal of Health and Social Behavior* 4:179-83.

Gluckman, M. 1965. *The Ideas in Barotse Jurisprudence.* New Haven: Yale University Press.

Grob, G. 1983. "Disease and environment in American history." In Mechanic, D. (ed.), *Handbook of Health, Health Care and the Health Profession.* New York: Free Press. 3-22.

Haggerty, R. 1983. "Epidemiology of childhood disease." In Mechanic, D. (ed.), *Handbook of Health, Health Care, and the Health Professions.* New York: Free Press. 101-19.

Idler, E. 1992. "Self-assessed health in mortality: A review of studies." In Mares, S., Leventhal H., Johnson, M. (eds.), *International Review of Health Psychology.* New York: Wiley, 33-54.

Imboden, J.B., Canter, A., and Cluff, L.E. 1961. "Symptomatic recovery from medical disorder." *Journal of the American Medical Association* 178:1182-84.

Imboden, J.B., Canter, A., Cluff, L.E., and Trever, R.W. 1959. "Brucellosis III: Psychologic aspects of delayed convalescent." *Archives of Internal Medicine* 103:406-14.

Jahoda, M. 1958. *Current Concepts of Positive Mental Health.* New York: Basic Books.

Jones, K., and Vischi, T. 1979. "Impact of alcohol, drug abuse and mental health treatment on medical care utilization: A review of the research literature." *Medical Care* 17:Supplement.

Kaplan, G.A., and Camacho, T. 1983. "Perceived health and mortality: A nine-year follow-up of the Human Population Laboratory cohort." *American Journal of Epidemiology* 117:292-304.

Kassirer, J. 1992. "Clinical problem-solving: A new feature in the journal." *New England Journal of Medicine* 326:60-61.

Kleinman, A. 1988. *The Illness Narratives: Healing and the Human Condition.* New York: Basic Books.

_____. 1986. *Social Origins of Distress and Disease: Depression, Neurasthenia and Pain in Modern China.* New Haven: Yale University Press.

Langner, E.J., and Rodin, J. 1976. "The effects of choice and enhanced personal responsibility for the aged: A field experience in an institutional setting." *Journal of Personality and Social Psychology* 34:191-98.

Larue, A., Bank, L., Jarvik, L., and Hetland, M. 1979. "Health in old age: How do physicians' ratings and self-ratings compare?" *Journal of Gerontology* 34:687-91.

Leventhal, H. 1985. "Symptoms reporting: A focus on process." In McHugh, S. and Vallis, T.M. (eds.), *Illness Behavior: A Multidisciplinary Model.* New York: Plenum, 219-37.

Linn, B.S., and Linn, M.W. 1980. "Objective and self-assessed health in the old and the very old." *Social Science and Medicine* 14:311-15.

Maddox, G.L., and Douglass, E.B. 1973. "Self-assessment of health: A longitudinal study of elderly subjects." *Journal of Health and Social Behavior* 14:87-93.

McHugh, S. and Vallis, T.M. 1985. *Illness Behavior: A Multidisciplinary Model.* New York: Plenum.

Mechanic, D. 1990. "Promoting Health." *Society* 27:16-22.

_____. 1988. "Social class and health status: An examination of underlying processes." *Conferences on Socio-economic Status and Health.* Palo Alto, CA: Henry J. Kaiser Family Foundation.

_____. 1986a. "Illness behavior: An overview." In McHugh S. and Vallis, T.M. (eds.), *Illness Behavior: A Multidisciplinary Model.* New York: Plenum, 101-09.

_____. 1986b. "Some relationships between psychiatry and the social sciences." *British Journal of Psychiatry* 149:548-53.

_____. 1986c. "The role of social factors in health and well being: The biopsychosocial model from a social perspective." *Integrative Psychiatry* 4:2-11.

_____. 1983. *Handbook of Health, Health Care, and the Health Professions.* New York: Free Press.

_____. 1982a. "Disease, mortality, and the promotion of health." *Health Affairs,* 1:28-32.

_____. 1979. "Correlates of physician utilization: Why do major multivariate studies of physicial utilization find trivial psychosocial effects." *Journal of Health and Social Behavior* 20:387-96.

_____. 1978. *Medical Sociology: A Selective View,* 2d ed. New York: Free Press.

Mechanic, D. (ed.), 1982b. *Symptoms, Illness Behavior and Help-Seeking.* New Brunswick: Rutgers University Press.

Mechanic, D., and Angel, R. 1987. "Some factors associated with the report and evaluation of back pain." *Journal of Health and Social Behavior* 28:131-39.

Mechanic, D., and Hansell, S. 1987. "Adolescent competence, psychological well-being and self-assessed physical health." *Journal of Health and Social Behavior* 28:364-74.

Mechanic, D., and Newton, M. 1965. "Some problems in the analysis of morbidity data." *Journal of Chronic Diseases* 18:569-80.

Mechanic, D., Cleary, P.D., and Greenley, J.R. 1982. "Distress syndromes, illness behavior, access to care and medical utilization in a defined population." *Medical Care* 20:361–72.

Mossey, J.M., and Shapiro, C. 1982. "Self-rated health: A predictor of mortality among the elderly." *American Journal of Public Health* 72:800–8.

Osterweis, M., Kleinman, A., and Mechanic, D. (eds.), 1987. *Pain and Disability: Clinical, Behavioral and Policy Perspectives.* Committee on Pain, Disability and Chronic Illness Behavior, Institute of Medicine. Washington, DC: National Academy Press.

Phillips, D., and Feldman, K. 1973. "A dip in deaths before ceremonial occasions: Some new relationships between social integration and mortality." *American Sociology Review* 38:678–96.

Phillips, D., and King, E.W. 1988. "Death takes a holiday, mortality surrounding major social occasions." *Lancet, ii.* 728–32.

Rodin, J. 1986. "Aging and health: Effects of the sense of control." *Science* 233:1271–76.

Rodin, J., and Langner, E.J. 1977. "Long term effects of a control-relevant intervention with the institutionalized aged." *Journal of Personality and Social Psychology* 35:897–902.

Spitzer, W.O., and Task Force 1986. *Rapport du Groupe de Travail Quebecois sur les Aspects Cliniques des Affections Vertebrales Chez les Travailleurs.* Quebec: L'Institute de Recherche en Sante et en Securite du Travail du Quebec.

Syme, S.L. 1986. "Social determinants of health and disease." In Last, J. (ed.), *Maxcy-Rosenau Public Health, Health and Preventive Medicine,* 12th ed. Norwalk, CT: Appleton-Century-Crofts.

Tessler, R.C., and Mechanic, D. 1978. "Psychological Distress and Perceived Health Status." *Journal of Health and Social Behavior* 19:254–62.

Tornstam, L. 1975. "Health and self-perception: A systems theoretical approach." *The Gerontologist* 27:264–70.

Verbrugge, L., and Ascione, F.J. 1987. "Exploring the iceberg: Common symptoms and how people care for them." *Medical Care* 25:539–69.

Waitzkin, H. 1991. *The Politics of Medical Encounters: How Patients and Doctors Deal with Social Problems.* New Haven: Yale University Press.

Ware, J.E., Jr. 1986. "The assessment of health status." In Aiken, L.H. and Mechanic, D. (eds.), *Applications of Social Science to Clinical Medicine and Social Policy,* New Brunswick, NJ: Rutgers University Press, 204–28.

White, K. 1970. "Evaluation of medical education and health care." In Lathem, W. and Newberry A. (eds.), *Community Medicine: Teaching, Research and Health Care.* New York: Appleton-Century-Crofts, 274.

White, K., Williams, F., and Greenberg, B. 1961. "The ecology of medical care." *New England Journal of Medicine* 265:885–92.

5

Promoting Health and Independence

The U.S. Department of Health and Human Services (HHS) has completed a long and detailed process in developing national health promotion and disease prevention objectives for the year 2000. This process, involving twenty-two expert working groups, the health departments of the various states, almost 300 national organizations and some 10,000 participants, resulted in an ambitious agenda organized under twenty-two major general objectives such as physical activity and fitness, nutrition, maternal and infant health, violent and abusive behavior, unintentional injuries, and so on. With each of these areas, there are three types of objectives: those pertaining to achieving a certain level of health status; those involving risk reduction; and those relating to services and protection. Many of these objectives are extrapolations of possible achievements relative to base rates, without specification of the data base that make these targets realistic or strategies of how specific goals can be achieved.

The process of establishing objectives, and involving influential national groups in efforts to achieve them, is a highly significant activity. However, the nation also needs a clear conception of an implementation process and the range of realistic initiatives that might be taken to achieve these goals. One important component of such a plan is a theoretical conception of how change can best be encouraged and the relative role of individual action, community mobilization, and social policy.

The Challenge

Health promotion has become very fashionable. In a recent major conference, speaker after speaker reiterated the need for more attention to improved life-styles, particularly in such areas as smoking, drinking, nutrition, and exercise. The session then adjourned to dinner festivities, where little else was available but liquor and beer, salted snacks, and a variety of bratwursts. This instance would be unworthy of comment except that it typifies the enormous gap between our rhetoric and our behavior and helps identify the challenge that serious efforts at health promotion must face. The point is simple but crucial; most behaviors, either conducive or detrimental to health, are influenced as much or more by the routine organization of everyday settings and activities as they are by the personal decisions of individuals. Health education efforts that ignore this fact are destined to failure.

American society places high value on health, as reflected in public attitudes, the more than $800 billion a year expended on health services, and the immense interest reflected in the media. Since the 1970s, there has been a growing health consciousness, and there have been efforts made to induce an increased sense of personal responsibility for physical fitness and improved behaviors in areas relevant for health, in part motivated by the uncontrollable escalation of medical care costs. Whether considering educational campaigns relevant to cigarette smoking, alcohol and drug use, or those devoted to exercise, nutrition, and safety, it is evident that health promotion has become a growth industry. The AIDS epidemic, and its close link to personal sexual and drug-using behavior, reinforces the shared view that individuals play a major role in their own destinies and can shape their vitality, health, and longevity.

The Importance of Group Structures

Effective health promotion requires scrutiny of the structure of communities and the routine activities of everyday life, as well as stronger interventions than those characteristic of much that goes on. Current efforts still function largely at the margins. Almost a hundred years ago, Emile Durkheim published his classic study of suicide, in which he examined how social constraints characteristic of varying groups and situations were linked with suicide rates. He identified two processes associated with suicide but in somewhat different ways. First, a loosening of social constraints, whether characteristic of egoistic suicide or anomie, was associated with elevated suicide rates. Alternatively, a high level of social integration associated with a tradition of ritualistic suicide in response to duty could also lead to high rates.

Durkheim's insights on how group structures constrain individual behavior are important for developing appropriate strategies for change. The strength of the individual's ties to the immediate social context determines the scope of influence exercised over behavior. As the level of social integration diminishes, the group—whether family, neighborhood, or larger social entity—is less successful in enforcing its expectations. When group commitment and social integration are strong, the specific norms characteristic of the group and its normal settings shape the boundaries of permissible behavior.

Most of the behavior we view as health-relevant is embodied in daily structures and routines. The regularity of daily functions, eating and sleeping habits, and routine exercise and levels of exertion, is substantially programmed for us. The norms of our social contexts define the appropriateness of a wide range of risk behaviors as well as the circumstances under which such behavior is permitted. Expectations and the shame of nonconformity impose standards for our efforts and motivate our achievements. These very basic group structures and processes account for much of the behavior we observe.

Active and Thoughtful Consumers

As attention focused on health promotion, researchers sought to identify behavioral orientations particularly conducive to positive health behavior. These efforts were disappointing, because behavior relevant to health resulted from a variety of motives, many of which had little to do with health. While there were clusters of behaviors moderately associated with one another (i.e., cigarette smoking, alcohol use, use of marihuana), the clusters had low correlations with one another, and occasionally were even negatively associated.

The research literature gives us little reason to anticipate isolating a health promotion inclination that can be used as a vehicle to change behavior across a broad spectrum of activities. Alternatively, however, we can identify important social characteristics that contribute positively to a range of health-promoting activities. Health behaviors seem to be influenced more by culturally and socially rewarded adaptational styles than by specific health motivations. Consistent positive health behavior results from its integration into complex repertoires of behavior that are sustained by interlocking networks of reinforcements. Thus, the route to promoting health may be approached through the broad processes by which education, culture, and religious and moral obligations are advanced.

The Constraints of Culture

In his book, *Who Shall Live?*, Victor Fuchs (1974) explains the huge differences in death rates between the contiguous states of Utah and Nevada by the fact that "Utah is inhabited primarily by Mormons, whose influence is strong throughout the state. Devout Mormons do not use tobacco or alcohol, and in general lead stable, quiet lives. Nevada, on the other hand, is a state with high rates of cigarette and alcohol consumption and very high indices of marital and geographical instability" (p. 53). As Fuchs points out, the states are comparable on many of the indices associated with mortality, such as income and schooling. They share many other similarities, as well, such as climate, urbanization, and concentration of health care resources. Fuchs is correct in a general sense, but Mormonism and its influence encompass a variety of features that not only affect health indices but also are related to low rates of delinquency, crime and violence, high educational achievement, and a purposeful orientation. In these respects, Mormons are not unlike other cultural groups such as Jews, Chinese, and Japanese, who also perform well on many health and other social indices.

Mormons and other groups with good health indices share a strong kinship structure that serves as a solid base for childhood socialization, a positive orientation to education, and an ethic that gives work a meaningful place in the group's value structure. The Mormon church teaches the importance of the family, parenthood, and family relationships, and encourages a strong orientation toward mastery of the environment, emphasizing active effort, accomplishment, and the acquisition of skills and education. As Thomas O'Dea notes in his book, *The Mormons*,

Life is more than a vocation, more than a calling; it is an opportunity for deification through conquest, which is to be won through rational mastery of the environment and obedience to the ordinances of the church. This doctrine, permeating individual and community life, is expressed today in a configuration of attitudes clustering around activity and development. This configuration represents an important aspect of the individual's integration into the life of the Mormon group, for it relates the striving of individuals to collectively prescribed ends. Moreover, since it is taught by exhortation and example from early childhood, this set of attitudes becomes second nature to those brought up in the Mormon home and community environment. (O'Dea 1957:143-44)

Mormons have good health not simply because they value health and refrain from smoking and drinking. Mormon health derives in part incidentally from the daily routines that evolve out of the accepted patterns of everyday living, including family, work, and play.

The presence of a well-knit group structure that demands a person's loyalty and commitment is only an enabling factor. Also at issue are the particular values, goals, and preferences that are taught and rewarded. Early studies on medical care utilization that focused on ethnic groups in New York City found that ethnic exclusivity and cohesiveness resulted in greater skepticism of medical care. But a similar study among Mormons found that a comparable group structure may encourage high acceptance and use of medical services. Group structures provide a basis for influence. But the content of values shapes behaviors.

The Role of Education

Education is the single most important predictor across a broad range of health outcome measures. Education, however, is an extraordinarily complex variable that is related to information acquisition and processing, styles of life, self-conceptions, patterns of work and recreation, coping strategies and many other aspects of behavior and interpersonal associations. Schooling of the mother, in particular, affects infant survival; the growth, health, and vitality of the child; and the child's developmental trajectory (Caldwell 1986). Children of better educated parents do better in school and advance further in their own educations than children of comparable ability of less well educated parents. It has been suggested that the schooling of parents is a proxy for the complexity of the home environment and the extent to which the child receives mental stimulation and learns complex coping skills (Spaeth 1976). Persons with more education seek out information more aggressively, and understand and retain more of it. Schooling, thus, is a significant enabling factor for promoting health.

It remains unclear, however, whether the effects of education on health are primarily due to its cognitive aspects, or more to the way education structures preferences, social and cultural orientations, ways of life, and coping skills. Inkeles (1983), for example, has argued that a behavioral orientation, which he calls "psychological modernity," is essential for the development of societies, but studies of psychological modernity suggest that most of its effects are explained by schooling. As Inkeles observes, the process of schooling itself requires students to develop behaviors that are essential for modern productive societies, such as following a schedule, keeping appointments, and learning from the modeling of others. Persons with more schooling are open to new experiences, are more likely to question authority, are more ambitious, engage in planning, and are more inclined to participate in civic and community affairs. In short, schooling energizes persons to more actively engage their environments. Such persons are more interested in and less fatalistic about their health, seek out more health information, and are more likely to view health problems as within their control.

Levels of Intervention

The forces—economic, social, and personal—leading to behaviors harmful to health are pervasive and influential. These behaviors may be immediately gratifying to those who engage in them, and major international industries such as those involved with tobacco and alcohol have an important stake in encouraging high levels of consumption. Enormous sums are invested in advertising and other promotional schemes that encourage practices detrimental to health. In comparison, health-promotion efforts are feeble attempts with relatively few resources to counteract noxious influences. Combining strategies in mutually reinforcing combinations may provide stronger opportunities for effective countervailing influence. Such efforts need to be pursued at the individual, community, and social policy levels.

We often work on the assumption, despite knowing better, that if we provide the public with appropriate information on behaviors favorable or detrimental to health, the power to determine their health futures is within their control. Health educators do not believe that information itself produces the desirable behaviors, but it is typically believed that information when combined with motivated behavior will produce the targeted outcomes. There is now considerable research showing that at least three elements are essential to induce various health behaviors: knowledge of the positive value of a particular behavior; motivation to adopt the behavior whether induced by fear or by some other energizing influence; and a plan designating the steps by which the behavior can be implemented (Leventhal, Prohaska, and Hirschman 1985). This third aspect, involving the coping element of the behavioral response, is usually neglected because it is assumed that most people know how to perform the desired behavior. However, when implementation is broken into its smaller elements, it becomes clear that there are many barriers or interferences with behavior implementation, and that perhaps the most difficult aspect of behavior change is providing people with workable strategies for dealing with these barriers (Leventhal 1982).

Behaviors also vary substantially in the extent to which they require continued motivation or vigilance. In the case of discrete behaviors involving single actions, such as getting a particular immunization, there is much less challenge to public health officials than there is in sustaining the continuing motivation necessary in such complicated longitudinal behaviors as exercise, maintaining a proper diet, or taking appropriate protection during sexual activity. In each of these instances, and in many others, public health efforts must be geared not only to initiating complex behaviors but to sustaining them over time through realistic reinforcements.

Some examples will make these points more clear. Throughout much of the world there is large concern with adolescent sexual behavior, adolescent pregnancy, and the threat of AIDS. Major campaigns are being launched to encourage youngsters who are sexually active to use condoms to protect against both AIDS and unwanted pregnancy. An analysis of adolescent sexual behavior would suggest that sexual behavior is not planned, but rather is part of a complex set of interpersonal transactions that are viewed by the youngsters as evolving spontaneously. Indeed, much of the appeal in these transactions may come from the gaming rituals that take place, the unplanned character of the interaction, and the uncertainty of the outcome. Many youngsters have no idea of how to disrupt this sequence in an acceptable or unembarrassing way to insure that appropriate protection is arranged. Successful health promotion in this area requires considerable instruction on how to gracefully interrupt this type of behavioral sequence or to prepare for it. This is difficult to do, and explains our relatively limited success in changing high-risk sexual behavior among adolescents.

Or consider the case of a youngster who is aware of the dangers of alcohol abuse, and would prefer not to drink, but who also desperately wants the approval of peers. He or she finds themselves in a situation in which not only peers are drinking but in which they put considerable pressure on the youngster to join them as part of group social activity. This is a threatening situation for many youngsters, particularly those with low self-esteem and limited coping capacities, and many are at a loss to understand how to resist such pressures without loss of status. These dilemmas are quite common and often present barriers that block the enactment of well-intentioned motivated behavior.

Successful health promotion requires not only motivating persons to practice health-inducing behaviors, but also restructuring norms and the ordinary settings of daily life at work and home to make implementation of desired behaviors more possible. To the extent that healthful behaviors are built into our daily routines and are socially valued, the behaviors will occur regularly without us giving much thought to them. In contrast, behavior based on conscious decision making requires continuing vigilance to overcome the inevitable barriers that arise, and, thus, such behavior is inherently more unstable. If my daily work routines require me to walk five miles during the day, such exercise occurs without my thinking about it. If I have to plan each day to find some time for daily exercise, its occurrence depends on the success of my scheduling, determination in adhering to the regimen each day, and the absence of events that will disrupt my plans. While some planning for health behavior will be essential in all of our lives, ultimate success will depend on the extent that we can successfully integrate health behaviors into the routine organization of daily life.

Family Influence

The family is a key institution in facilitating the integration of health-promoting routines into one's daily life, although this area has received relatively little analysis in the health-promotion literature. It has been recognized for some time that marriage, particularly for men, is associated with lower levels of mortality (Mechanic 1978), probably due in part to the constraints of family routines. More recently, Umberson (1987) found that both marriage and parenting were associated with less health damaging behaviors. While marriage had stronger effects for men than for women, the effects of parenting were similar and were only operative when children were actually present in the home. These, and other findings, suggest the importance of health structuring within the family. Women, however, are more likely to regulate health-related behavior within families (Umberson 1990).

It remains unclear how health regulation in families functions, although a variety of alternative possibilities seems to be available. These include scheduling, joint activities, interfamily facilitation, interpersonal monitoring, encouragement, routinization, and reinforcement. Family life sets important constraints on everyday activities by prescribing when certain events are to take place, such as meals, morning rising, sleep, weekend activities, and the like. Particularly where children are involved, parents must organize their lives so that children eat, are properly groomed, get to school on time, and so on. These responsibilities set constraints on when parents must be available, their sleeping and rising habits, and the amount of regularity in daily routines. There is, of course, great variability in how families function, but, on average, well-functioning families are characterized by reciprocal influence processes.

Interfamily facilitation of positive health behavior can operate in many ways, including joint activities. Family meals allow regulation of diet, and opportunities to encourage regular eating patterns and good nutrition. Use of alcohol is either moderated or encouraged by the behavior of spouse and other family members, and common drinking patterns appear to be more frequent than chance. Families may put time aside for exercise together or for completing chores such as gardening that encourage activity. Joint activities have demand characteristics and help overcome lapses in personal motivation.

Implicit in many of these activities is encouragement of good health practices, common in parenting and in spouse relationships. Family members are in strategic positions to monitor health-related practices of other family members and to encourage positive health behavior not only for the individual but for the family as a unit. Examples include the effects of cigarette smoking on nonsmoking family members, effects of smoking and drinking during pregnancy, careful driving and use of seat belts, etc. Monitoring and encouragement can work in many directions, as when children who learn about the noxious consequences of smoking in school encourage their parents to quit. Families also provide a context for continuing reinforcement of positive health behavior.

Family Influences on Adolescence

Families have a major influence on the development of children and adolescents and the patterns of behavior they adopt. Even in circumstan-

128   Inescapable Decisions

ces of little income and education, children in strong families that encourage education, effort, accomplishment, and environmental mastery do well. Good health outcomes seem to be linked inextricably with positive outcomes more generally. Conversely, those subgroups with the poorest health outcomes also have high rates of school dropout, delinquency, premarital pregnancy, and disrupted family life.

In a longitudinal study of over a thousand adolescents in nineteen public schools in New Jersey, my colleague Stephen Hansell and I (Hansell and Mechanic 1990) sought to identify how parental and peer value systems affected health-relevant behavior across seven types of behavior, including alcohol use, cigarette smoking, marihuana use, seatbelt use, sports activities, other exercise, and eating breakfast. We proceeded on the assumption that adolescents were socialized simultaneously within two value systems, one oriented toward family and parents, the other toward peers. These two systems of values could be more or less congruent, although parents are more likely to emphasize long-range goals and consequences while same-age peers generally focus on enjoyment of the present and experimentation.

Adolescents vary in the extent to which they adopt parental values, depending on family cohesiveness and other factors. Most parents place high value on the efforts and skills necessary for enhancing future life chances of the adolescent and commonly urge the adolescent's attention to the long-term consequences of current behavior. In comparison, adolescent subcultures place major value on peer-oriented social activities and immediate gratification. Many studies show that adolescent peer activities typically expose adolescents to, and commonly encourage them to engage in, cigarette smoking, substance abuse, and other risk-taking behaviors.

We used proxy measures to represent adolescents' commitment to these two value systems. Proxies for adherence to a parental value orientation included perceptions of parental interest, having dinner with parents, good academic grades and attendance at religious services. In contrast, we measured the influence of peer orientations by an index of peer social activities including hanging around with friends, talking with friends on the phone, and going to parties. We anticipated that identification with parental values would relate positively to health behavior across a range of dimensions, while adherence to peer values would have negative effects.

The longitudinal results provided strong support for our hypothesis that higher engagement in parent-oriented activities was associated with positive changes across diverse health behaviors. Eating dinner with parents and religious attendance were associated with a number of improvements in health behavior over time, but perceived parental interest and academic grades were particularly important in accounting for positive changes in health behavior. We also found that adolescents more strongly involved with peers were consistently more likely to engage in risk behaviors over time. Such peer involvement significantly increased smoking, alcohol, and marihuana use over time. Peer interactions, of course, provide important socialization experiences relevant to adolescent development and well-being. But many studies also suggest that peer groups encourage risk-taking and often place low value on academics and other parent-oriented cultural values. Effective socialization in families earlier in life persists in its influence, even after young adults have left the family and spend most of their time in association with peers (Lau, Quadrel, and Hartman 1990). A major challenge is to modify the culture of adolescent peer groups toward constructive values and activities, and effective families can affect this process. The integration of youth groups into a system of broad and constructive values and goals is a powerful vehicle for positive health change.

The literature in general, and data from our studies more specifically, suggest the importance of children's perceptions of parental interest and concern. Even as adolescents strike out to assert their independence and autonomy, they depend substantially on the security of a caring family. But caring, however important, is not sufficient unless it is linked with achievable but high expectations (Bock and Moore 1986). Effective adaptation requires that young persons acquire the needed motivation, skills, and coping capacities to carry out required tasks and to relate appropriately to other people. Young people develop a sense of mastery and esteem by taking on meaningful responsibilities and by contributing in a constructive way to their families and communities. Challenges must be manageable and not overwhelming, but dealing with challenge is a prerequisite for the development of effective behavior.

The Nature of Health Knowledge and User-friendly Markets

What we mean by health knowledge may seem obvious, but on closer inspection it remains problematic. At issue is the amount of knowledge necessary for effective healthful behavior, and the likely accessibility of that knowledge to most people. For example, we tell people that they should eat a healthy and nutritious diet and particularly counsel them on cholesterol consumption, the appropriate balance between fat, carbohydrates, and protein, and the importance of roughage. Even when individuals understand the recommended instructions, ambiguous or misleading labeling of food products makes it difficult to follow expert advice, except in the most general ways.

Perhaps, even more important is that food consumption occurs increasingly outside the home, and it is difficult for consumers to know how the food they eat is prepared, or whether "health foods" that are widely promoted in response to consumer interests, are really healthy. As the consumer movement grows it may be possible to modify how fast food and other restaurant products are prepared, or the range of choice, but such changes will be as much a product of politics and marketing decisions as of an individual's decision to follow a healthy diet. Difficulty is compounded by the fact that the public is given many, and often conflicting, health messages. These messages may conflict on the facts, as in prevalent information now made available concerning cholesterol reduction, or the messages may change over time. People readily become aware of these contradictions and confusions, and many health messages lose their credibility. Given the complexities of information flow, the massive amounts of information available to the public, and scientific uncertainty, it is inevitable that sorting through health messages requires judgment and effort.

What we seek, thus, is an active and thoughtful public that can process information, an information environment that is reasonably coherent and user friendly, and community norms and patterns of activity that reinforce behavior conducive to good health outcomes.

Changing Culture

The forces affecting health behavior, like those affecting behavior more generally, are complex and multifaceted. As previously noted, to the extent that such behavior is programmed into the culture and everyday activities of a group, the behavior is more likely to be reliably performed. Similarly, to the extent that social settings are structured to be conducive to positive health, people will face fewer barriers in the implementation of favorable intentions. But changing culture and the structure of social settings are formidable tasks, and such change occurs only slowly and usually not without social and political opposition. Processes of culture change require collective action and depend on the principles by which social movements become established and innovations diffused among populations. The process itself has several interrelated elements. First, there has to be an agenda—a set of ideas and practices that are seen as conducive to some valued goal. Second, there have to be credible innovators who serve as models for the adoption of the desired practices. Third, there has to be some motivating force, shared by the larger target population, that encourages taking up new practices. And fourth, there have to be reinforcers that sustain a new practice until it becomes part of the natural flow of everyday activities.

In many instances, there may be strong inducers and reinforcers working against change. Many of the behaviors detrimental to health are immediately rewarding, are often sustained by powerful economic interests that promote the noxious practice, or are so integrated into current cultural practices that they are repeatedly reinforced, often inadvertently, and are strongly resistant to change.

Smoking constitutes a reasonable success story, particularly in the context of the intense advertising efforts of the industry. It is impossible to untangle the influences that reduced smoking, but it is clear that the culture has changed, as has individual behavior. Smoking has been prohibited in many public places and restricted in public transportation, in restaurants, and in workplaces. Perhaps even more important is the fact that the norms have been modified sufficiently to put smokers on the defensive. It is no longer embarrassing to ask people not to smoke in social settings, and smokers are increasingly made to feel apologetic about their behavior. Such normative changes may not induce many people to give up smoking but will probably change the frequency and context of smoking, making it easier for those who want to quit. Even more important, young people are growing up in contexts in which they sense growing disapproval of smoking, and this may work as a deterrent to initiating the behavior.

Other types of behavior, such as alcohol consumption, are so much a part of social occasions that there are strong inducers to drink even among those inclined not to. Drinking is inevitably associated with occasions of conviviality and recreation and serves as a lubricant for socialization.

The patterning of alcohol use at parties, taverns, athletic events, and the like makes it inevitable that drinking and driving will be associated. While such devices as collecting car keys at teenage parties or using designated drivers for partying groups may help at the fringes, the organization of social life still induces and sustains drinking and driving.

What has been briefly noted about smoking and drinking can be said about almost any common behavior detrimental to health. Such behaviors flourish in contexts that routinely sustain them and usually require vigilance and conscious choice to resist. The challenge is to define points of leverage that change the balance of influences so that everyday activities favor more positive patterns. This requires coordinated programs that make efforts that are regulatory, technological, and educational.

Our culture generally resists regulation of personal choice. It is clear that the ease of access affects use. Self-service machines for cigarettes make them more accessible to youngsters; the age at which drivers can obtain a license affects rates of injury and death; taxes on alcohol and cigarettes affect levels of consumption. In any instance, while there may be reluctance to prohibit access, regulatory alternatives for restricting accessibility still remain viable options. These restrictions are likely to have their largest effects on youth, a point that raises the issue of targeting.

Targeting Interventions

One strategy is to target efforts to yield the largest possible result. There are several possible target objectives. First, it is valuable to target young people before they acquire health destructive habits that are difficult to modify. Although such targeting involves a large potential audience, it may be easier to prevent an initial behavior such as smoking, drug use, or risky sexual behavior than change it once it becomes established within the individual's behavioral repertoire. Moreover, young people can be approached through school and after-school programs that make preventive efforts more feasible and less expensive. A second type of targeting is on the behavior itself. The view persists that if children can be taught effective decision making it can affect a broad range of behaviors, and many school health programs are not focused. Since many of the behaviors most deleterious to health are not highly correlated, it seems reasonable to specifically target those behaviors that are associated with the greatest health risk, such as smoking. Third, it makes sense to focus resources on the subgroups of the population that have the highest known probabilities of exposure to risk. Too many health-promotion programs address populations that are most receptive, and typically these populations are at least risk and probably least likely to require a special intervention.

In high-risk populations, the barriers to implementation are commonly quite extensive, and programs need to give considerable attention to the plan for coping, the usually neglected element of the health message. Strategies for reinforcing health instruction, using peers, teachers, parents, and media help sustain the instruction over time. The potential influence of such instruction depends on the extent that parents and peers are complementary influences and the degree to which a peer group subculture can be developed that is reinforcing of the positive behavior.

One important way of supporting good health practice independently of conscious positive health behavior is to incorporate it into the technology itself. We are all familiar with inflatable air bags and involuntary seat belts, the safe cigarette, low-salt food products, fireproof garments, and the like. Such technical solutions to risk depend on cost and consumer acceptability. Much more could be done to develop technologies that promote health as well as potential markets for such products. Industry is extraordinarily adaptive in responding to consumer wants; encouraging the development and expansion of health-promoting products and activities should be part of any long-range strategy.

The Potential of Health Promotion

In many instances, health promotion is a feeble effort relative to the incentives and reinforcements that encourage health-destructive behaviors. Expenditures to promote smoking among susceptible and vulnerable populations, relative to our meager counterefforts, highlight the political nature of the health-promotion challenge. More typically, however, the forces producing behavior detrimental to health are insidious and ubiquitous in our daily lives. They relate to how we organize work and recreation, our eating patterns and how we prepare food, our sedentary styles of activity, the social uses of alcohol, our increasing dependence on cars and door-to-door transportation, and many more. Many of these behaviors are rewarding, and contribute to perceived quality of life and, thus, are difficult to change without significantly modifying preferences.

It is not at all clear that health values are or should be paramount or that we should seek to alter rewarding behaviors simply because they are not optimal for health. Stress may be discomforting, but it also often contributes to effort and achievement. Moderate drinking may assist social relations and add a spark to social intercourse. Some sports are dangerous but also exhilarating. Many foods high in fat and sugar are particularly enjoyable. The automobile is especially convenient, and few consumers are willing to trade this for a cleaner environment or a lower probability of accidents and injuries. In short, health promotion has to offer a vision of healthful alternatives that are equally attractive to those behaviors we ask the public to give up.

I suggest that one reason persons of higher socioeconomic status more readily adopt positive health behavior than those more disadvantaged is that they have more daily gratifications that can substitute for the gratifications one gets from smoking, drinking, or overeating. In the most disadvantaged groups, or among persons under stress, the tension reduction associated with smoking, drug use, and alcohol may be more gratifying than a future health benefit. Health promotion works best among people who feel a great stake in their futures and who therefore value the long-deferred benefits of current behavior. Many adolescents and disadvantaged people have yet to perceive the type of stake that motivates giving up immediate gratifications.

How, then, do we build conceptions of alternative futures, scenarios associated with less morbidity and greater longevity but also with a gratifying life-style? I believe one does this by developing cultural consensus and group-supported values that make healthy life-styles attractive and rewarding. We also do it by improving living conditions so that all subgroups have hopeful prospects and a stake in the future.

References

Bock, R.D., and Moore, E.G.J. 1986. *Advantage and Disadvantage: A Profile of American Youth*. Hillsdale, NJ: Lawrence Erlbaum Associates.

Caldwell, J.C. 1986. "Routes to low mortality in poor countries." *Population and Development Review* 12:171–220.

Fuchs, V. 1974. *Who Shall Live?: Health, Economics, and Social Choice.* New York: Basic Books.

Hansell, S., and Mechanic, D. 1990. "Parent and peer effects of adolescent health behavior." In Hurrelmann, K. and Lösel, F. (eds.), *Health Hazards of Adolescence.* Berlin: Walter de Gruyter, 43–65.

Inkeles, A. 1983. *Exploring Individual Modernity.* New York: Columbia University Press.

Lau, R.A., Quadrel, M.J., and Hartman, K.A. 1990. "Development and change in young adults' preventive health beliefs and behavior: Influence from parents and peers." *Journal of Health and Social Behavior* 31:240–59.

Leventhal, H. 1982. "The Integration of emotion and cognition: A view from the perceptual motor theory of emotion." In Clarke, M. and Fiske, S. (eds.), *The Seventeenth Annual Carnegie Symposium on Cognition.* Hillsdale, NJ: Lawrence Erlbaum Associates, 121–56.

Leventhal, H., Prohaska, T.R., and Hirschman, R.S. 1985. "Preventive health behavior across the life span." In Rosen, J.C. and Solomon, L.J. (eds.), *Prevention in Health Psychology.* Hanover, NH: University Press of New England, 191–235.

Mechanic, D. 1978. *Medical Sociology,* 2d ed. New York: Free Press.

O'Dea, T.F. 1957. *The Mormons.* Chicago: University of Chicago Press.

Spaeth, J.L. 1976. "Cognitive complexity: A dimension underlying the socioeconomic achievement process." In Sewell, W.H., Hauser, R.M., and Featherman, D.L. (eds.), *Schooling and Achievement in American Society.* New York: Academic Press, 161–76.

Umberson, D. 1990. "Marital status and the regulation of health behavior." Paper presented at the Annual Meetings of the American Sociological Association, Washington, DC

_____. 1987. "Family status and health behaviors: Social control as a dimension of social integration." *Journal of Health and Social Behavior* 28:306–19.

6

Socioeconomic Status and Health

One of the most enduring relationships in all of social science is the association between social class and a wide array of measures of mortality, morbidity, well-being, and use of health services. Lower social status is predictive of fetal wastage and perinatal death, infant mortality, developmental problems, morbidity, psychological distress, and longevity (Mechanic 1978; Susser, Watson, and Hopper 1985; Mechanic 1982; Last 1986; Aiken and Mechanic 1986). While these associations are well recognized, there is lack of clarity about the causal processes and the relative importance of intervening factors. In this chapter, I examine a variety of conceptual, methodological, and substantive issues that relate to underlying processes and possible hypotheses for meaningful health interventions.

The Concept of Social Class

Social class is typically used in sociology as a central theoretical concept indicating the individual's location in the social stratification system and access to material resources, influence, and information. This concept may be used in a highly theoretical way, as in Marxian analysis, with precise structural implications, but it is more commonly used as a descriptive indicator denoting a variety of recognized cultural and economic attributes that can be scaled in a variety of ways. In empirical analysis it is often useful to disaggregate the components of social class, but theoretically, the concept is intended to capture in a holistic way the meaning, within defined communities, of occupying a particular social location and its implications, not only for material welfare but also for

137

prestige, networks of association, community influence, and cultural styles.

Qualitative studies of community stratification map the sociocultural implications of class differences, but most quantitative studies use a limited number of indicators: income, education, occupation, and occasionally, residence. These are important not only in terms of their direct implications, but also because they are substantially associated with a wide range of other factors that affect people's health, well-being, and life chances. In some instances, social class and its specific components have direct causal influence on health factors; in others, the association is spurious, resulting from influences associated with both health and social class.

Indicators of social class only imperfectly capture its theoretical meanings, and the indicators themselves may vary across historical periods and cultures (Sewell 1982). This problem is reflected, for example, in debates concerning the effects of poverty, because income deprivation is a *relative concept* and the absolute material resources of the poor in our society may exceed those of many of the world's population, who would not so identify themselves. Similarly, the significance of a year of education, or total education attained, depends both on its meaning in a particular cultural context and the average level of education in a society overall. It would be foolish to equate the attainment of a college education among cohorts born in 1920 and 1960. Both the content and the cultural meanings change over time. Various studies of occupational prestige, however, show such prestige to be relatively invariant over time (Hodge, Siegel, and Rossi 1964), although there are clear shifts in the educational and income attributes associated with particular occupations.

The changing attributes of the labor market and occupational structures are intensively researched. The details need not concern us here. Crucial for the discussion that follows is the fact that descriptive statements between class indicators and health outcomes are bound by the time and context in which these observations are made. For example, prior to 1966, the poor used fewer physician visits and hospital bed days than the more affluent, but this relationship shifted following the introduction of Medicare and Medicaid. The limitations of descriptive findings for identifying generic interventions may be obvious, yet inappropriate generalizations from descriptive studies limited to particular periods and contexts are common. In the Medicare/Medicaid example, the intervening proximal determinants of the relationship—economic and physical access to services—are obvious, but as we examine more complex class and health linkages the underlying processes are more difficult to disentangle.

A Note on Measures of Socioeconomic Status

The major indicators of socioeconomic status are substantially inter-correlated in most populations, but each may have differential influence in varying instances. Researchers attempting to capture a more complex picture of social class may seek to develop comprehensive indices of socioeconomic status, but they do so at some cost. Education, income, occupation, and residence may each have different effects on specific dependent variables, and these effects may vary as well, depending on labor force participation (Kessler 1982). Given increasingly sophisticated multivariate methods, the availability of large data sets, and the power of modern computers whenever possible, it is advantageous to disaggregate index components to examine their unique effects and interactions with other measures. Thus, for example, Kitagawa and Hauser (1973) demonstrated that education and income have independent effects on mortality, and Kessler (1982) showed that income, education, and occupational status all have independent effects on levels of psychological distress.

The Meaning of Social Class Indicators

Indicators of social class are commonly associated with cultural practices, family life, child-rearing practices, self-conceptions, community involvements, cognitive skills, and coping strategies. They are predictive as well of quality of housing, nutrition, access to medical and social services, recreation, and many other goods and services. Since the number of linkages is extraordinarily large, it is useful to think of class effects in terms of some generic categories. By doing so we can better understand linkages and also intraclass variance.

Class can be seen as affecting exposure to environmental risk, opportunities to access valued material resources and information, the development of cognitive schema, cognitive complexity and coping skills, and access to social networks and instrumental support. Class also has important influence on self-conceptions and problem-solving orientations, as well as values and interests. Each of these factors may bear directly on health behavior and health status or may be associated rather loosely with particular life trajectories that have many complex transition points. Choices and decisions made at varying points in the life cycle involving marriage, pregnancy, termination of schooling, and job affect the probabilities of later life chances. Class also may affect the propensity to "drift" into particular trajectories in contrast to careful information acquisition and planning. Social position of one's family at birth substantially affects the probabilities of varying life trajectories. In the remainder of the chapter, I illustrate some of the processes and suggest some implications for interventions. But, first, some methodological caveats.

Threshold Effects and Social Selection

It is common to observe that much of the observable health impact occurs below a certain threshold of social status and that once certain levels of income, education, and job status are reached, additional effects are more modest (Mechanic 1978). Hundreds of studies show that poor health, inappropriate health behavior, and social pathologies cluster significantly in the lowest socioeconomic groups, with high rates of most types of pathology in these social strata (Robins 1979, 1983). It is debatable whether it is appropriate to view these populations as part of an underclass, but it is important conceptually to differentiate such populations, which are relatively small, from all others who may be in poverty at any point in time.

Poverty is a time-limited status for a majority of the poor; within this population are subgroups characterized by long-term poverty, profound health and social risk, high levels of demoralization and anomie, and highly prevalent illness, mortality, and violence. Since most available data are cross-sectional, it is extraordinarily difficult to track how this more intractably poor population differs from the transient poor. It is difficult to link appropriately the necessary data sources, since even large representative surveys of the population do not sample sufficient numbers of the population at highest risk to allow substantial analysis. This population at highest risk is also difficult to survey, requiring us to depend to a greater degree than we would like on limited studies.

A closely associated issue involves the assortative processes that result in low socioeconomic status. In many instances, low social status is a consequence of biological vulnerability, poor health status, and social pathology, and in most data sets it is impossible to identify the direction of influence. Moreover, selection effects occur through a variety of processes including assortative mating, residential drift, and job selection, complicating our understanding of the biological and behavioral predictors. How individuals come together, live together, marry, have and raise children are difficult to model, but these selective processes have influential effects on the health of children, their psychological and social development, and their future life chances.

Social Status and the Physical Environment

Socioeconomic status affects exposure to noxious aspects of the physical environment through its influences on residence and occupational risks. Substantial numbers of deaths and injuries occur in the workplace, and risks are significantly higher in blue-collar occupations and among unskilled laborers. Such risks include accidents, as in mining and construction, or high levels of exposure to noxious substances, as in the manufacture of chemicals. There are at least nineteen chemicals or industrial processes for which there is reasonably convincing epidemiological evidence of carcinogenicity in humans, including asbestos, benzene, vinyl chloride, and chromium. Many others are highly suspect but involve less definitive evidence (Brandt-Rauf and Weinstein 1983:272). Other sources of danger clearly associated with disease or disability include: coal dust and tars, hot and cold temperatures, cotton dust, noise, and high exposure to metals such as lead, manganese, and tin.

Environmental hazards are found in the indoor environment, food, water, waste and sewage, and in contamination of the air. Crowding, deficient appliances, poor maintenance of housing structures, and low quality of household equipment and ventilation all may contribute to risk through accident, fire, or environmental degradation. Although I pass over this important area quickly, it should be apparent how each of the socioeconomic status (SES) indicators noted earlier is likely to affect these risks through both voluntary and involuntary behavior. Better educated persons are more likely to know the risks, can make choices that are in part informed by such awareness, and can take other preventive actions. Economic resources provide access to safer homes and neighborhoods, allow purchase of better functioning appliances and house maintenance, and give more choice of neighborhood. Residents in higher socioeconomic areas are better able to protect themselves by zoning and other political processes from traffic and other sources of exposure, not only to noxious contaminants but also to crime and other potential dangers. While SES is not the only or even the major source of exposure to environmental risk, it constitutes a significant part of the picture.

Persons in higher socioeconomic groups are less likely to be unable to work because of disability than those lower in the social hierarchy. This reflects both differences in exposure to risk contributing to disability and the fact that physical deficits are much more limiting in jobs at the lower levels of the occupational structure. While professional and technical personnel and clerical workers are greatly underrepresented among the disabled population, farm and service workers, laborers, and workers in the crafts are significantly overrepresented (Rest 1986:905). Disability is also influenced, in part, by motivation: the greater prevalence of disabled at the lower ends of the occupational spectrum reflects the fact that disability benefits are more comparable to wages at lower income levels.

In considering occupational and environmental risk, much of the variance is explained by the specific risks inherent in particular work and living situations, irrespective of social status. Thus, physicians have high risk of drug abuse, influenced by their easy access to addicting drugs, and nurses have a high prevalence of lower back injury specific to the types of work they do. However, because the highest risks of noxious exposure and injury tend to be associated with jobs at the lower ends of the occupational spectrum and because housing conditions and neighborhood quality are closely linked with income, the socioeconomic effects in the aggregate are substantial. Nevertheless it is unlikely that we have much to learn by pursuing these aggregate relationships in contrast to targeting specific risks associated with specific jobs.

Social Class and Occupational Attainment

From a health viewpoint, there are at least two reasons to examine briefly the literature on social class and occupational attainment. First, as a highly developed area of research (Blau and Duncan 1967) it suggests causal processes that have bearing on the questions we ask about health. Second, occupational attainment and its correlates, as we have already noted, are an important factor in health outcomes.

The Wisconsin model of status attainment is perhaps the best-developed single model and is consistent with the results of most other major studies that are less comprehensive (Sewell and Hauser 1975). The study, based on the cohort of all high school seniors in Wisconsin in 1957, included follow-up observations in 1964 and acquisition of tax records in 1965 to assess earnings. The analysis conveys the complexity and specificity of mobility processes, suggesting caution to workers in the health arena about the scope of generalization. While the Wisconsin model was highly successful in explaining educational achievement, accounting for 54 percent of the variance, it accounted for only 43 percent of the variance in occupational attainment and 7 percent of the variance in 1967 earnings. The latter result reflects in part the fact that earnings in the sample had not stabilized by 1967, but also that many factors other than the determinants of educational attainment influence earned income.

The Wisconsin model indicates that the most important influences in obtaining higher education are the decision to plan to go to college and college entry itself. Both socioeconomic origins and ability are powerful predictors of such planning and decision making. While only approximately half of high-ability boys and a quarter of high-ability girls of lower SES origins in the cohort studied enrolled in college, 90 percent of high SES boys and 76 percent of high SES girls of comparable ability enrolled. These influences persist through graduation. Only 38 percent of low SES/high-ability boys graduated compared with 71 percent of high SES/high-ability boys. Comparable figures for girls are 50 and 67 percent. Thus, while ability was important in selecting students for higher education, SES continued to be a major determinant of the selection process.

In modeling educational and occupational attainment, important intervening variables include high school performance, encouragement of educational and occupational aspirations by significant others, and the aspirations students develop, which in turn depict processes most influenced by background factors. Additional factors unrelated to ability or socioeconomic origins influence the levels of encouragement and aspirations. Socioeconomic status does not affect performance in high school independent of ability, but it strongly affects educational and occupational attainment through the influence of significant others. The ability of the student, in contrast, independently affects both high school performance and the encouragement students receive from significant others, which in turn predict educational and occupational attainment.

While SES is a powerful force in these attainment processes, much of the variation is not explained by SES, ability, and other intervening factors. This is as it should be, since many influences contribute to attainment, such as motivation, personality, capacity for sustained effort, and luck. The complexity of these processes is worthy of some emphasis, since it realistically depicts what we should expect to find in examining SES and health outcomes. Logically, genetic health endowment, although more difficult to measure, is comparable in health models to the ability indicator in status attainment models. It would be useful to attempt to objectify more clearly what every physician takes into account in taking a medical history—the individual's biological health stock. But the key point is that many factors other than SES or health endowment affect the intervening variables that modify health outcomes, and if we are to target interventions effectively, the challenge is to identify better those intervening variables more proximal to the health outcomes of special interest to us.

Social Class and Cognitive and Behavioral Processes

Socioeconomic status is moderately associated with measures of intellectual ability. I would like to sidestep the acrimonious debate as to how much of this correlation can be explained by the character of ability tests as compared with social selection effects. Persons of less ability, as we have seen, have lesser educational and occupational attainments, and substantial marriage assortment occurs to bring such persons together. The evidence also demonstrates, however, that high levels of educational attainment occur in the absence of high ability when other factors are promotive.

High levels of education facilitate the acquisition of knowledge and skills, as well as the development of cognitive capacities. Similarly, certain types of work are likely to facilitate how people think about their environment and how they solve problems. Thus educational and oc-cupational attainment are likely to be important for coping, independent of the ability of individuals or the tangible and intangible rewards educational and occupational attainment bring.

Kohn and Schooler (1978) have observed that intellectual flexibility, self-direction, and greater well-being are associated with job conditions that involve more complex substance, are free of close supervision, and are nonroutine. In contrast, job considerations that lack these characteristics promote a conformist orientation. In an intriguing presentation, Spaeth (1976) argues that much of the status-attainment process could be understood in terms of the transmission of the capacity to cope with cognitive complexity. He argues that

> statuses relevant to socioeconomic achievement can be considered as indicators of the complexity of settings to which persons are exposed. In the family of orientation, children may not only be exposed to complex stimuli; but parents may also manipulate those stimuli; serve as role and competency models and bring about treatments that increase (or decrease) the competency of their children in coping with cognitive complexity. (P. 130)

In support of his interpretive framework, Spaeth finds that the correlation between occupational complexity (as measured by Kohn) and occupational prestige is .8, which in turn is correlated .6 with schooling. He views schooling as a measure of exposure to increasingly complex educational environments, and parental SES as a proxy for the complexity of the child's cognitive environment. Parental SES is associated with a wide variety of environmental attributes, including talking and playing with the young child, talking to the child during meals, and providing explicit instructions and positive feedback (Spaeth 1976:108). As Schooler (1972) has suggested, the child exposed to a more complex environment is better able to cope intellectually with complex and ambiguous situations.

Status attainment, like health behavior and health status, is best thought of as a series of contingencies, none of which completely determines the outcomes. In extending this line of thinking, Miller, Kohn, and Schooler (1986) found that schooling reproduces high socioeconomic status through "differential training of independent, self-directed orientations in students." Through initiative and independent judgment, cognitive functioning becomes enhanced.

The implications of this large body of research are intriguing. Education, for example, is one of the most consistent predictors of measures of mortality, morbidity, and health behavior. It is also associated with smaller family size and parental interest in the child (Mechanic 1980). It seems plausible to anticipate that parents with higher levels of interest and knowledge about health and those with greater interest in their children will be more likely to make investments for the health of their children, will create healthful environments for their children's development, and will provide more direct health instruction consistent with maintaining health.

It seems plausible, in addition, that educational attainment is a proxy for such diverse factors as rearing practices, attitudes and values, parental interest and nurturance, coping instruction, self-esteem, and opportunities to invest in health, but there is no empirical model available that explains the effects of education in a coherent way. Despite some serious measurement difficulties, Pratt's research on the influence of family structure on health behavior (Pratt 1971) points to coping competence as a key consideration. Pratt found that both education and family structure were associated with health behavior, but when the latter was taken into account, education had no further net effects. She argues that

> men and women whose family arrangements provide opportunities for autonomy and personal growth are more likely to assume full personal responsibility for caring for their own health, to seek out the best methods of health care, to strive for maximum development of their physical capabilities, and to be resourceful in responding to the changing health needs of their bodies. (Pratt 1976:86)

Pratt, unfortunately, does not present a sufficiently developed model to assess varying effects. In an effort to examine Pratt's hypothesis, I found some evidence in support of the importance of self-esteem and certain family processes on health behavior, but these were mostly independent of education (Mechanic 1980).

Social Class, Health Values, and Health Knowledge

Social class is substantially related to values, interest in health, knowledge about health matters, and preventive health actions (Feldman 1966; Mechanic and Cleary 1980). It also affects how persons respond to illness, how they express their problems and health concerns, how they retain information and services, and how they cooperate in treatment. The literature in this area is large but highly descriptive and not very analytical. In general, education has the largest effects among class indicators on health knowledge and values, but the relative importance of education, occupation, and income depends on the specific issue under consideration. Education, for example, is most influential in the acquisition and retention of information, whereas income is often important in issues involving access to and retention of services.

Kohn (1977), in his theory of occupational self-direction noted earlier, provides the single most coherent approach to his topic. His basic thesis is that the relationship between social class and values derives from underlying conditions of life characteristic of different positions in the social structure. He emphasizes the substantive complexity of work and self-direction as his core concern, but these concepts may apply equally well to home environments and leisure pursuits. Kohn presents considerable evidence indicating that middle-class parents value self-direction, whereas working-class parents put larger emphasis on conformity to external authority, and these attitudes in turn influence disciplinary practices as well as relative parental responsibilities in setting constraints for children. This approach suggests that children raised in environments emphasizing self-direction will be more likely to develop their intellectual and coping capacities and acquire a stronger sense of self. Kohn does not directly give much emphasis to health, but he has argued that the conditions of conformity characteristic of the working class restrict coping flexibility and put vulnerable children at risk when they are under stress. While the process Kohn posits is plausible, the links between class and the outcomes of major interest are not well developed.

On a descriptive level, education is substantially associated with greater knowledge and a greater inclination to acquire further knowledge. As Feldman (1966) has noted, those less educated are not only less informed, but also are less exposed to new information and appear to learn less when exposed. Thus knowledge and ignorance perpetuate themselves (Feldman 1966:56). It is for this reason, he maintains, that health education makes only slow progress in reaching less-informed groups. It remains unclear how much educational differences reflect varying ability and openness to information in comparison with differential access. Certainly there is extraordinary informational access in American society. Few studies probe deeply enough to examine whether the varying levels of information characteristic of groups with different levels of education reflect varying exposure to and ability to understand health messages, or whether persons in varying classes differ in their capacities or inclinations to update their health knowledge over time.

Consideration of Kohn's theory in relation to descriptive data on acquisition of health knowledge suggests the hypothesis that persons of lower education are more likely to acquire health information in a prescriptive way, while those with higher levels of education are more inquiring, more open to new information, and more proactive in upgrading and updating what they know. The difference between health information and knowing how to acquire it is an important one, because the possible stock of health knowledge is very large and changing and most people have limited need for most of it. Thus it seems important for people to have search strategies to alert them when further information is necessary and skills to acquire it. Many studies suggest that in illness behavior situations, the most common alerting factor is a change from expected or customary levels of function. The seriousness of such changes is often judged by the extent to which they interfere with goals and usual activities, and not by medically relevant criteria. These decisions are arrived at through a "commonsense" self-assessment. To the extent that a medical definition of danger is preferable, it becomes necessary to program individuals to bypass usual commonsense explanations in assessing meaning.

Assessment of Ecological Data

Most of the findings discussed involve surveys and epidemiological investigations, but much data of interest come from correlating attributes of populations, such as the proportion who are black with rates representing these populations. Associations from such ecological analyses tend to be higher than those from data sets involving individuals and also to be more difficult to interpret clearly. Typically, income and educational characteristics of census tracts or statistical reporting areas are substantially associated with a wide range of indicators of poor health, deviant behavior, and family disorganization.

Such ecological correlations depict the culmination of a variety of selection and causative processes impossible to disentangle in such data. Ecological areas with high rates of pathology compound the noxious environmental, housing, family, and personal influences that contribute to health problems. These areas also provide the only living contexts for those who failed in a variety of social roles. Thus there are often disproportionate numbers of single-parent families, unemployed individuals, homeless individuals, decarcerated mental patients, and criminals, etc. Such data, thus, can serve as no more than clues for further investigation. By themselves they are unlikely to take our understanding much further.

Conclusion

Socioeconomic status is linked through a variety of pathways to many important influences on life trajectories. It is perhaps the single most important influence on health outcomes, in part through its direct influence, but, more importantly, through the many indirect effects it has on factors that directly shape health outcomes. Socioeconomic status thus serves as a window that helps identify important points of intervention and remediation. It is, of course, desirable to improve economic security and educational attainment, but practicality requires that we also identify factors more closely associated with health outcomes so that we maximize opportunities to intervene effectively. In either case, socioeconomic status remains an important focus for promoting future health.

References

Aiken, L., and Mechanic, D. (eds.), 1986. *Applications of Social Science to Clinical Medicine and Health Policy.* New Brunswick, NJ: Rutgers University Press.

Blau, P.M., and Duncan, O.D. 1967. *The American Occupational Structure.* New York: Wiley.

Brandt-Rauf, P.W., and Weinstein, I.B. 1983. "Environment and disease." In Mechanic, D. (ed.), *Handbook of Health, Health Care, and the Health Professions.* New York: Free Press.

Feldman, J. 1966. *The Dissemination of Health Information.* Chicago: Aldine.

Hodge, R.W., Siegel, P.M., and Rossi, P.H. 1964. "Occupational prestige in the United States, 1925-63." *American Journal of Sociology* 70:286-302.

Kessler, R. 1982. "A disaggregation of the relationship between socioeconomic status and psychological distress." *American Sociological Review* 47:752-64.

Kitagawa, E.M., and Hauser, P.M. 1973. *Differential Mortality in the United States: A Study in Socioeconomic Epidemiology.* Cambridge, MA: Harvard University Press.

Kohn, M. 1977. *Class and Conformity: A Study in Values,* 2d ed. Chicago: University of Chicago Press.

Kohn, M., and Schooler, C. 1978. "The reciprocal effects of the substantive complexity of work and intellectual flexibility: A longitudinal assessment." *American Journal of Sociology* 84:24–52.

Last, J. (ed.). 1986. *Maxcy-Rosenau Public Health and Preventive Medicine*, 2d ed. Norwalk, CT: Appleton-Century-Crofts.

Mechanic, D. 1982. "Disease, mortality, and the promotion of health." *Health Affairs* 1:28–32.

_____. 1980. "Education, parental interest and health perceptions and behavior." *Inquiry* 17:331–38.

_____. 1978. *Medical Sociology*, 2d ed. New York: Free Press.

Mechanic, D., and Cleary, P.D. 1980. "Factors associated with the maintenance of positive health behavior." *Preventive Medicine* 9:805–14.

Miller, K.A., Kohn, M.L., and Schooler, C. 1986. "Educational self-direction and personality." *American Sociological Review* 51:372–90.

Pratt, L. 1976. *Family Structure and Effective Health Behavior: The Energized Family*. Boston: Houghton Mifflin.

_____. 1971. "The relationship of socio-economic status to health." *American Journal of Public Health* 61:281–91.

Rest, K. 1986. "Problems in special groups." In Last, J. (ed.), *Maxcy-Rosenau Public Health and Preventive Medicine*, 12th ed. Norwalk, CT: Appleton-Century-Crofts.

Robins, L. 1983. "Continuities and discontinuities in the psychiatric disorders of children." In Mechanic D. (ed.), *Handbook of Health, Health Care, and the Health Professions*. New York: Free Press.

_____. 1979. "Follow-up studies of behavior disorders in children." In Quay, H.C., and Werry, J.S. (eds.), *Psychopathological Disorders of Childhood*, 2d ed. New York: Wiley.

Schooler, C. 1972. "Social antecedents of adult psychological functioning." *American Journal of Sociology* 78:299–322.

Sewell, W.H., Jr. 1982. "Occupational status in nineteenth-century French urban society." In Hauser, R.M., Mechanic, D., Haller, A.O., and Hauser, T.S. (eds.), *Social Structure and Behavior*. New York: Academic Press.

Sewell, W.H., Jr., and Hauser, R.M. 1975. *Education, Occupation, and Earnings*. New York: Academic Press.

Spaeth, J.L. 1976. "Cognitive complexity: A dimension underlying the socioeconomic achievement process." In Sewell, W.H., Jr., Hauser, R.M., and Featherman, D.L. (eds.), *Schooling and Achievement in American Society*. New York: Academic Press.

Susser, M., Watson, W., and Hopper, K. (eds.). 1985. *Sociology in Medicine*, 3d ed. New York: Oxford University Press.

PART III

Special Populations

7

Adolescents at Risk

As I look at the growing field of research on adolescents at risk, I am impressed that research efforts have yet to catch up with what I will call commonsense conceptions of adolescence and young adulthood. The commonsense position is that children who grow up in decent neighborhoods and well-integrated families, and who have parents and other close role models who communicate interest, caring, and support, but who also convey high but realistic expectations and standards, are substantially protected against significant risks associated with the adolescent developmental period.

The research on individual risks, of course, identifies many specific antecedents for each area of concern, and any broad effort to encompass such varied arenas of behavior will be simplistic to some degree. The specific antecedents of sexual promiscuity are quite different from those of interpersonal violence or abuse of alcohol, and efforts to identify general personal orientations or personality types that are generally predictive of risk-taking have been disappointing. This may be an entirely wrong approach and one that even if it was more successful would confront us with the extraordinary impediments of changing ingrained, difficult-to-modify personal behavior.

A contrasting approach is to identify the specific contextual conditions that contribute to family and community disorganization and increase the probability of adolescent risk behavior, and examine the alternatives available to modify them or to ameliorate their effects.

Let me begin with certain generalizations that I believe to be consistent with the research literature. Children and adolescents are highly resilient. Moreover, as historical and cross-cultural experience make clear, normal development is consistent with an extraordinary range of household and family structures and sociocultural variations. Poverty and family disorganization increase the probability of deviance, but most children and adolescents growing up in poverty or in disrupted households progress normally and do not develop significant pathologies. Even in extreme cases of potential harm, where parents are highly deviant, abuse alcohol and drugs, and mistreat their children—perhaps the sources of highest risk—a significant proportion of these children demonstrate good adaptive capacities and resilience.

Social development is extraordinarily complex, and no single factor will be explanatory. What we typically see is a matrix of events over time in which particular adversities increase the probability of subsequent risk events. Brown and his colleagues in England, for example, have suggested that early loss of mother substantially reduces the probability of adequate child and adolescent care (Harris, Brown, and Bilfulco 1987). Young girls, perhaps anxious to escape oppressive and unhappy homes, become prematurely involved in relationships. Having less than adequate coping skills for dealing with these relationships, they are more likely to experience premarital pregnancies and enter unsuitable marriages. These lead to subsequent difficulties that increase vulnerability to adult depression and other undesirable outcomes. The broader point is that many of the problems of concern are part of a developmental trajectory in which events of interest are dependent on earlier influences and choices that affect subsequent options. Choices about schooling, jobs, marriage, childbearing, and their timing establish the conditions for future choices and outcomes (Brown 1986).

The events in the scenario described above are linked to social class. In each case, social class influences the intervening variables that contribute to risk, but class itself is unlikely to play a major direct causal role. Social class, for example, affects the capacity and resources of the single parent to provide adequate caring for young children, and the limited resources associated with poverty may give the adolescent few opportunities to develop alternative gratifications or coping skills and confidence to avoid early sexual relationships and pregnancy.

Social class is important because it potentially affects a very broad range of important influences, including access to knowledge, material resources, self-esteem, personal mastery, cognitive complexity, and many others (Mechanic 1989). Poverty, in the absence of other family or cultural strengths, can substantially reduce life chances and contribute to a sense of alienation and hopelessness. Reducing poverty is clearly one direct way of intervening in high-risk life trajectories (Bunker, Gomby, and Kehrer 1989), but it is not in itself sufficient.

The literature gives enormous attention to the emotional climate of the family and the quality of interest and caring in relation to the child and adolescent. It is well established that adolescence is a time of increasing self-awareness and one in which youth test their autonomy and independence. It is also a time when peer group pressures compete seriously with family influences, and adolescent peer groups have a high propensity toward risk activities involving alcohol and drugs, sex, cars, and the like. At the same time, peer activities teach interpersonal and other coping skills important to social development. Our impression from our work with adolescents and young adults is that they depend substantially on the security of home and parents even as they strike out for independence and autonomy. Their ability to do this is aided by their sense that parents are truly interested in them, care deeply about their welfare, and would come to their assistance if needed.

Love and acceptance are clearly not enough. Young people, if they are to make satisfactory adaptations, have to develop the necessary motivation, skills, and coping capacities to obtain and carry out jobs and relate appropriately to other people. These skills are important assets in the transition to adult life and set the stage for much that follows. There is now widespread concern about the long-term erosion in academic capacities of young people and the implications of these trends for the quality of the U.S. work force. No one seems very clear on why the intellectual and physical skills of U.S. youth have declined, nor why U.S. youth now lag behind those in most other developed countries. It may be that the materialism that pervades our culture, and the lack of commitment to deeper goals, dampens motivation beyond acquisition of material items. Thirty or forty years ago, adolescents who worked did so as a means to contribute to the family as a struggling economic unit, as do many adolescents from Asian and other immigrant communities today. Many adolescents continue to have part-time jobs, but the proceeds are more frequently devoted to the purchase of cars and the latest stereo equipment than to the economic viability of the family (Greenberger and Steinberg 1986).

There is some research supporting the view of thoughtful observers that young people mature and develop a sense of efficacy and esteem through assuming meaningful but manageable responsibilities. Elder (1974), for example, studied a cohort of children who grew up during the Depression. Working-class children and their families faced major adversities, and many of these children had problems later in life. The prevalence of such problems was probably due to the overwhelming nature of the deprivations faced by many of these working-class families. Middle-class children, in contrast, who faced deprivations were more symptom-free in adulthood than their counterparts who were more sheltered. Of the nondeprived middle class, 26 percent had behavior disorder problems in adulthood as compared with 7 percent among those experiencing deprivation. Heavy drinking in adulthood was much more common in the nondeprived middle class (43 percent versus 24 percent). One can suggest a variety of alternative hypotheses to explain these results, but one plausible notion is that manageable deprivations that demand responsibility from the adolescent contribute to the development of coping capacities and self-respect, major assets for the future.

The foregoing suggests two alternative pathways to developmental problems. The first refers to deprivations of large magnitude that overwhelm adolescents and their families and result in hopelessness and a failure to see possibilities and alternatives. This, I believe, may be the plight of many of the so-designated underclass in our ghettos, confined to deteriorating neighborhoods, devastated by crime, poverty and substance abuse. Single-parent families with inadequate income and limited educational and coping resources provide a highly problematic environment for growing up. The prevalent street subculture in these areas, and the web of street associations, lead youth toward substance abuse, crime, violence, and risk-taking. Moreover, unlike middle-class youth, these adolescents are probably less likely to have "second chances" once they get into difficulty.

Alternatively, many U.S. youth grow up in environments that are economically secure but that make few demands for responsible contributions and mature behavior. These adolescents waste enormous amounts of time "hanging around" or being alone, typically passively watching television (Csikszentmihaly and Larson 1984). It is significant that these youth commonly report such activities as meaningless and boring, and not enjoyable. More important, they are losing innumerable opportunities to contribute to meaningful activities, to develop useful habits, to acquire effective coping skills, and to develop a deeper sense of self-respect and mastery.

Work on stress and coping suggests persuasively that adaptation is an active continuing process, in which challenges are stimuli for the development of effective behavior. Effective youth do not relate to their environment passively; they approach their lives in a purposeful way, anticipating challenges relative to their aspirations and goals, planning their agendas, rehearsing problems, considering alternative solutions, and seeking relevant information (Mechanic 1986). As Silber (1961) and his colleagues reported in a study of competent adolescents, "The active search for manageable levels of challenge in newness is more characteristic of the coping behavior of competent adolescents than a stabilized adaptation to the environment with maximal reduction of tension," (p. 265). Similarly, Seligman (1975) has argued that many problems in adult life result from removing challenge during important developmental stages. A sense of worth and self-esteem, he believes, can only be earned. He argues, "If we remove the obstacles, difficulties, anxiety, and competition from the lives of our young people, we may no longer see generations of young people who have a sense of dignity, power and worth," (p. 159).

The issue is not middle-class affluence but how this affluence is used. In the aggregate, affluence gives youth enormous advantages in access to a more complex preschool environment; to high-quality schooling; and to a broad range of social, cultural, and intellectual opportunities. Thus, social class, and particularly parental education, consistently predicts effective performance, good health outcomes, and psychological well-being. Affluent youth have more opportunities in an array of school and extracurricular activities and more chances to develop skills in musical and artistic performances, in theatrical groups, in team sports, in clubs, and in skill-demanding hobbies of all kinds. Affluent parents also contribute immensely to the life chances of their children irrespective of ability. At every point of educational selection, affluent children of no greater ability than less affluent ones do substantially better in reaching the next step (Sewell and Hauser 1975).

The massive literature on the effects of social stratification on life chances and health make it clear that youngsters who grow up in poverty must overcome innumerable obstacles. Even in respect to schooling, which is fundamental for every child, students from lower socioeconomic strata receive less encouragement for their aspirations and less tangible assistance as they go through the schooling experience.

Many of high ability fall behind early, become discouraged, and drop out before attaining basic skills necessary to function. In ghetto environments, the problem is exacerbated by a neighborhood subculture that devalues academic performance and personal persistence.

As noted earlier, some youth prosper under what may seem horrendous conditions, and others do badly despite all possible advantages. Many factors are relevant including biological strengths and vulnerabilities, extraordinary social supports, and luck. Developmental trajectories are in no way inevitable regardless of initial conditions. This is nicely illustrated by a series of studies by Quinton and Rutter (1984a, 1984b) that examined the outcomes of girls who were under care of local authorities as children in England with a comparison group. In adulthood, these girls had high rates of early pregnancy, were less likely to be in stable cohabiting relationships, and had more difficulty taking appropriate care of their children. They had more difficulty than those in the comparison group in relating to their children and in showing warmth and sensitivity, and were more likely to be hostile. However, when these women had a supportive spouse, they did as well as those in the comparison group. But those with a history of local authority care were more likely to link up with a deviant partner and showed less planning in their relationships and marriages.

Defining a research agenda that focuses on the major points of leverage for intervention trials is no easy matter. How one intervenes to build the personal commitment of youth to shared goals, and provides them with the necessary adaptive skills, is one of the central challenges for any society (Panel on Youth 1974). There is now great interest in revitalizing the quality of schooling at all levels, but it should be evident that schools, no matter how outstanding, cannot achieve the desired goals through their own efforts. Two elements external to the quality of schooling itself—parental interest and involvement and peer culture—help shape the meaning of school and student involvement in it. Yet, research is needed to identify how best to enlist the needed supportive structures that facilitate the schooling process. Three ideas already discussed—family involvement, the power of expectations, and contextual principles—shape the schooling process. In respect to the first, family life influences the motivations, values, and commitments relevant to skill acquisition and achievement. The second principle emphasizes the importance of family and community expectations on performance

(Bock and Moore 1986). The communication of serious, but realistic, expectations establishes opportunities and sets constraints. Third, the immediate social context, whether characterized by social advantage, or by a group subculture inimical to academic achievement and supportive of deviance, shapes response in many important ways. We have to learn how to better structure the social contexts of youth to facilitate more positive outcomes (Mechanic 1990).

The process by which such restructuring of social contexts occurs is often described by the clumsy term "empowerment," but this concept has considerable relevance. Some decades ago, the sociologist Robert Merton proposed a theory in which he suggested that deviant adaptations occur when individuals acquire goals and aspirations but lack the means to accomplish them (Merton 1957). In the ensuing years, the growth of mass communications, and particularly popular television programming, has probably communicated a sense of the affluent middle-class life-style to every home in America. And the discrepancies between what young people want and expect and their capacities, skills, and opportunities to attain them have probably widened.

Empowerment may be seen as a process in which individuals learn to see a closer correspondence between their goals and a sense of how to achieve them, and a relationship between their efforts and life outcomes. Many young people appear to lack goals or any clear sense of how to achieve the goals they have. The idea of empowerment is consistent with work in a number of research areas demonstrating the importance of such orientations as self-efficacy and learned helplessness (Rodin 1986; Seligman 1975).

A debate among scholars has continued for decades as to whether the seemingly maladaptive behavior of ghetto residents or the underclass reflects a "culture of poverty" or rational adaptations to the adversities and constraints of persistent poverty. The discussion focuses on certain behaviors that make getting and keeping a job uncertain, such as not being on time, failing to plan ahead, and types of demeanor that alienate others. Scholars who have studied adaptive orientations across cultures, a pattern described as "psychological modernity" (Inkeles 1983), emphasize the crucial importance of education in establishing the necessary skills, attitudes, and values. Education assists in reducing fatalism and passivity and encourages openness to new experience and a connection to the broader concerns of the community. One implication is that superficial approaches such as trying to teach youngsters to use condoms or "say no" to drugs will inevitably fail to achieve the desired objectives. The needs for intervention go much deeper and are more pervasive.

The optimal initiatives to redirect existing trends and to lessen risk among youth remain unclear. Certainly schooling at all levels must be invigorated, and teaching should be more valued and rewarded. We need better mechanisms for involving parents in their children's socialization and schooling, and in encouraging, educating, and supporting them in raising their demands and expectations of their children. At the same time, we must address the issue of the growing numbers of children in poverty and seek ways to ameliorate effects in the short run, while we deal with structural causes in the longer perspective.

In 1988, the Grant Foundation's Commission on Youth and the American Future recognized the extent to which an important segment of youth have been neglected, largely those who never go to college (William T. Grant Foundation 1988). Caught in a squeeze between a growing emphasis on credentials and an employment market that provides incomes too low to escape poverty and dead-end jobs that offer little prospect for improvement, many of these young people see little hope for a promising future. The large number of single parents in these marginal positions, heavily concentrated in the service sector, guarantee that large numbers of children will grow up in poverty (Ellwood 1988). Despite employment, these families often live tenuous existences, with incomes too high to be eligible for welfare entitlements but too poor to acquire health insurance and meet other basic needs. These problems, deeply embedded in our economy and welfare structure, have been a source of careful research but no social consensus on how best to address them.

The Grant Foundation Commission addressed a variety of ways that public and private cooperation, and the voluntary sector, could help give youth a larger stake in the community and in citizenship, building on community programs throughout the country that appear to work. The indicators are dismaying, reflecting low youth participation in community affairs and citizenship activities such as voting. The commission advocated expanded community opportunities to all young people through service opportunities and youth organizations. Even more importantly, their report emphasizes the need for expansion of education, training, and employment opportunities throughout the entire economy.

As much as we can talk about mature and responsible youth, it is of little avail if they lack opportunities to get a reasonable job and progress into adult roles with increasing possibilities for establishing stable work and family relationships.

Although the commission was wise in seeking to identify best practice, there is compelling need to better understand what really works in engaging the hardest-to-reach youth, and how they can be put on a more positive trajectory. As with programs in almost every sphere, the persons most easily reached are those least needing the experience and training. We often underestimate the intensity of infrastructure necessary to reach out to underserved populations (Coates and Maxwell 1990) and to sustain them in efforts to overcome many of the barriers to change. We will need rigorous action research to separate the truly promising initiatives from many suggested interventions lacking empirical support.

There are undoubtedly many valiant efforts in communities, but this is hardly enough. The magnitude and seriousness of the problem calls for vigorous leadership to impress the nation with the urgency of the issue and the importance of mobilizing efforts on many fronts to strengthen family life, to improve our schools, and to engage young people in responsible service roles to their community. Whether this should include revitalizing national service programs such as VISTA and the Peace Corps, as the Grant Commission suggests, or to put in place a system of compulsory national service as advocated by increasing numbers of observers remains unclear. Developing such mechanisms in a way mean-ingful to the large variety of youth with different motivations, back-grounds, and skills is a momentous undertaking that would require extraordinary planning, preparation, and funding, and the development of a very strong supervisory infrastructure. Successful implementation will require a national consensus and strong presidential and congres-sional leadership, as well as the active commitment of the private sector.

There is mounting concern that the United States is losing its place in the world and is increasingly in a weak competitive position relative to other nations. Reports abound on the failures of our schools, and the growing deterioration of our youth's basic skills. There is no more important resource than the quality of our youth and their ability and preparedness to assume their responsibilities in the years ahead. It is urgent that we expeditiously attack the wide range of problems that bear on this issue.

References

Bock, R.D., and Moore, E.G.J. 1986. *Advantage and Disadvantage: A Profile of American Youth.* Hillsdale, NJ: Laurence Erlbaum Associates.

Brown, G. 1986. "Mental Illness." In Mechanic, D., and Aiken, L. (eds.), *Applications of Social Science to Clinical Medicine and Health Policy.* New Brunswick, NJ: Rutgers University Press, 175-203.

Bunker, J., Gomby D., and Kehrer, B. (eds.). 1989. *Pathways to Health: The Role of Social Factors.* Menlo Park, CA: Kaiser Family Foundation.

Coates, D., and Maxwell, J.P. 1990. *Lessons Learned from the Better Babies Project.* White Plains, NY: March of Dimes Birth Defects Foundation.

Csikszentmihaly, M., and Larson, L. 1984. *Being Adolescent: Conflict and Growth in the Teenage Years.* New York: Basic Books.

Elder, G., Jr. 1974. *Children of the Great Depression: Social Change in Life Experience.* Chicago: University of Chicago Press.

Ellwood, D. 1988. *Poor Support: Poverty in the American Family.* New York: Basic Books.

Greenberger, E., and Steinberg, L. 1986. *When Teenagers Work: The Psychological and Social Costs of Adolescent Employment.* New York: Basic Books.

Harris, T., Brown, G., and Bifulco, A. 1987. "Loss of parent in childhood and adult psychiatric disorder: The role of social class position and premarital pregnancy." *Psychological Medicine* 17:163-83.

Inkeles. A. 1983. *Exploring Individual Modernity.* New York: Columbia University Press.

Mechanic, D. 1990. "Promoting Health." *Society* 27:16-22.

_____. 1989. "Socioeconomic status and health: An examination of underlying processes." In Bunker, J., Gomby, D., and Kehrer, B. (eds.), *Pathways to Health: The Role of Social Factors.* Menlo Park, CA: Kaiser Family Foundation, 9-26.

_____. 1986. "Distress and coping in late adolescence: Epidemiology, help-seeking and social adaptation." *From Advocacy to Allocation: The Evolving American Health Care System.* New York: Free Press, 177-89.

Merton, R. 1957. "Continuities in the theory of social structure and anomie." *Social Theory and Social Structure,* rev. ed. New York: Free Press, 161-94.

The Panel on Youth of the President's Science Advisory Committee. 1974. *Youth: Transition to Adulthood.* Chicago: University of Chicago Press.

Quinton, D., and Rutter, M. 1984a. "Parents with children in care 1: Current circumstances and parenting." *Journal of Child Psychology and Psychiatry* 25:211-29.

_____. 1984b. "Parents with children in care 2: Intergenerational continuities." *Journal of Child Psychology and Psychiatry* 25:231-50.

Rodin, J. 1986. "Aging and health effects of the sense of control." *Science* 233:1271-76.

Seligman, M. 1975. *Helplessness: On Depression, Development, and Death.* San Francisco: W.H. Freeman.

Sewell, W.H., and Hauser, R.M. 1975. *Education, Occupation and Earnings.* New York: Academic Press.

Silber, E. 1961. "Adaptive behavior in competent adolescents." *Archives of General Psychiatry* 5:354–65.

William T. Grant Foundation Commission on Work, Family and Citizenship. 1988. *The Forgotten Half: Pathways to Success for America's Youth and Young Families.* New York: W.T. Grant Foundation.

8

Deinstitutionalization of the Mentally Ill
Efforts for Inclusion

David Mechanic and David Rochefort

President John F. Kennedy first described his proposal for a national community mental health program in a special message to Congress on February 5, 1963. It was subsequently enacted as the Community Mental Health Centers (CMHC) Act of 1963. In his message, Kennedy set a quantitative target for this effort: a reduction by 50 percent or more of the number of patients under custodial care within ten or twenty years (Kennedy 1963). In reality, the process of "deinstitutionalization" proceeded even more quickly and more extensively than that. By 1975, the number of patients in state and county mental hospitals had declined by 62 percent from the time of the president's message (65 percent from the peak of 559,000 in 1955). Falling further still over the next decade, the institutional census contracted to 110,000 in 1985 (NIMH 1989) despite growth in the U.S. population and irrespective of the increasing number of mental hospital admissions over much of this period.

Rare, indeed, is it in social policy-making for measured accomplishments to outdistance stated goals. Almost as unusual is the degree of fervid enthusiasm—among mental health professionals, advocates, public officials, and members of the general public—that surrounded initiation of the community mental health movement, of which patient relocation was an essential strategy (Rochefort 1984). For many, the proposed redirection in mental health care represented both scientific and

---

This chapter is based, in part, on "Deinstitutionalization: An Appraisal of Reform," *Annual Review of Sociology* 16 (1990), published with permission of Annual Reviews, Inc.

humanitarian progress, a major "psychiatric revolution" to sweep away a dark age of institutional confinement (Grob 1987b). Cameron (1978) has described this mind-set as a new ideological consensus that functioned to provide the political energy and commitment necessary to move away from the existing system of hospital-centered care and its entrenched interests.

After some thirty-five years of programmatic experience, however, reactions to deinstitutionalization today are much less positive. Another ideological consensus may be emerging, one that identifies deinstitutionalization as one of the era's most stunning public policy failures. Critics underscore, especially, the incomplete development and inadequate performance of the supportive services that were meant to accompany patient discharge and patient diversion activities (Dear and Wolch 1987; *Newsweek* 1986; Torrey 1988). Some judge it time to return to a state hospital-based mental health system (Gralnick 1985). Emblematic of these currents is a letter to the editor of the *New York Times* by Democratic Senator Daniel Moynihan of New York (*New York Times* 22 May 1989). Pointing to the growing numbers of deranged homeless persons and the undersupply of community-based mental health care in New York City, Moynihan mused that President Kennedy might have set down his pen before signing the CMHC Act had he been able to foresee such outcomes.

The current controversy and large body of accumulated data make the time opportune for appraising the record of deinstitutionalization in the United States. Seeking to provide a comprehensive overview of its causes, nature, and consequences, this chapter addresses several questions pertinent to this sociological phenomenon. What sociohistorical forces—before, coincident with, and after Kennedy's community mental health legislation—gave rise to and facilitated the practice of deinstitutionalization? How far has deinstitutionalization progressed, and at what rates over time and for different geographical areas? What have been the effects of deinstitutionalization on patients and on the general society?

Roots of Reform

Deinstitutionalization offers a compelling case study of the complexities of modern social policy-making. Justly recognized as a major innovation in both the philosophy and the practice of mental health services delivery, the program evolved over decades and came to stand, for a brief while at least, as a high-priority agenda item at the highest level of government. Throughout, many influences were operative, including changing ideas and attitudes about the nature of mental illness and its treatment, biomedical advances, social research, professional currents, legal activism, and the emergence of a powerful political coalition in support of the mental health reform movement. Just as important, however, the deinstitutionalization experience also illustrates the manner in which forces and events belonging to different policy fields can interact to produce far-reaching, if often unplanned, outcomes.

Sources of Deinstitutionalization

An early impetus for deinstitutionalization derived from World War II and the changing ideologies and experiences associated with it. The environmental and egalitarian notions that developed during this period were related to the horrors of Nazism (Grob 1987b), and encouraged a strong conception of environmental determinism. The experience of psychiatrists during the war in dealing with neuropsychiatric problems during combat encouraged a preventive ideology and the translation of military psychiatric techniques to civilian practice. Moreover, the rejection of large numbers of men for the armed services for psychiatric reasons, and the increasing fiscal strain on state mental hospitals with growing patient populations, focused interest on a broader mental health strategy and a preventive ideology (Mechanic 1989).

Already by the 1950s, there was evidence that some mental institutions were changing administrative practices and beginning a modest process of deinstitutionalization (Bockoven 1972; Scull 1984). A major impetus came through the introduction, in the middle 1950s, of the phenothiazines, which made it possible for large institutions to modify administrative policies and to reduce coercive restraints. The new drugs helped control patients' most disturbing psychotic symptoms and gave hospital staff and families confidence in the potential of less coercive care and hopes of greater predictability of patients' behavior. At about the same time, the National Institute of Mental Health was developing a research and action agenda based on a belief in prevention and the social malleability of mental disorder. With its encouragement, research was undertaken in large hospitals documenting the deleterious effects of hospitalization on patients' functioning, motives, and attitudes (Goffman 1961; Belknap 1956), and such results supported the growing community mental health rhetoric. For the most part, however, the ideology was based on premises that were either undocumented or false (Mechanic 1989). But the mental health rhetoric had a life of its own and served as the basis for federal policy (Grob 1987a).

It is generally assumed that deinstitutionalization began with a vengeance during the middle 1950s with the introduction of new drugs. As we document later, the timing varied substantially by state, and deinstitutionalization was limited in the early years. During the period 1955 to 1965, public hospital populations decreased by only 1.75 percent a year on average (Gronfein 1985a). While hospitals were now more ready to return patients to community settings, they often had no place to send them and no basis for their support in the community.

Deinstitutionalization accelerated in the late 1960s and 1970s with the growth of the welfare state and with the reinforcement of an egalitarian, noncoercive ethic. By the late 1960s, lawyers socialized in the civil rights battles of the decade turned their attention to the rights of the mentally ill with an attack on civil commitment (Ennis 1972; Miller 1976) and the development of a legal theory supporting patient rights and the least restrictive alternative (Brooks 1974). With changing state statutes, it became increasingly difficult to commit patients to mental hospitals. The growth of welfare enabled the large-scale reduction of public mental hospital populations and provided large economic incentives to state governments to do so. Thus, it became easier to leave mental hospitals and more difficult to be committed.

Influence of Federal Policy

For one hundred years, since the growth of public mental hospitals in the early and mid-1800s, mental health policy in the United States was the domain of the states. With a series of national legislative enactments following World War II that helped foster community mental health and deinstitutionalization practices, the federal government became the prime agent of innovation and reform in public mental health care. It was to continue to play this role for some thirty-five years, until intergovernmental changes of the first Reagan administration reestablished the states' primacy in the design and control of local mental health services.

In addition to creating the National Institute of Mental Health, the National Mental Health Act of 1946 provided funding for the development of pilot community care programs in the states and for the training of mental health professionals. The Joint Commission on Mental Illness and Health was brought into being by Congress in 1955. Studies conducted under its auspices documented the far-reaching problems of mental health care in the United States, and the commission's final report articulated the case for wholesale system reform, including a redefined role for state mental hospitals as smaller, more intensive treatment sites.

Rounding out these unprecedented legislative activities in mental health was the Kennedy administration's Community Mental Health Centers Act, which sponsored the creation of a new type of community-based facility providing inpatient, outpatient, emergency, and partial hospitalization services, as well as consultation and education to other community organizations. By 1980, more than 700 CMHCs had been funded under the program, or roughly half of the 1,500 centers projected as needed for nationwide coverage (Foley and Sharfstein 1983). Other shortcomings of the program included a general lack of coordination between CMHCs and local state hospitals and a tendency among many centers to underserve the severely and chronically mentally ill (Dowell and Ciarlo 1989). CMHCs thus constituted more of a parallel than a complementary network of services to existing state care systems, yet the program did expand the alternatives to traditional institutions while promoting the community care ideology.

Beginning in 1966, and extending to the late 1970s, there was a rapid expansion of federal social welfare programs. Medicare and Medicaid, introduced in 1966, stimulated an enormous expansion of nursing home beds and provided an alternative for many elderly mentally ill and demented patients. Medicaid assumed the costs of care for patients moved from state institutions to nursing homes. Since states paid no more than half of Medicaid costs, they had strong incentives to shift patients to nursing homes, where the federal government would share the costs. In addition, the expansion of disability insurance made it much easier to return patients to family and board-and-care settings with sufficient income to contribute to their support. During this period there was also expanded public housing that provided housing opportunities directly, or indirectly, by adding to low-income housing stock. Thus, the expansion of the welfare state contributed to a stronger economic and residential base for deinstitutionalization. The depopulation of public mental hospitals accelerated, with patient populations decreasing an average of about 8.6 percent a year between 1965 and 1975 (Gronfein 1985a).

Contending Theoretical Explanations of Deinstitutionalization

Varying theoretical interpretations of deinstitutionalization arise from alternative conceptions of the role of the state in democratic capitalist society, from the degree of credibility given to the self-described objectives of key public actors, and from the phase of the policy-making process described.

One major approach analyzes the landmark community mental health legislation of the early 1960s, recognizing this as the occasion when deinstitutionalization became official national policy. This perspective emphasizes the idealistic and intellectual underpinnings of the community mental health movement, focusing on forces operative in the emergence, formulation, and approval of this legislative agenda. A spirit of melioration is seen as a driving force in the era's politics across a spectrum of issues from civil rights, to health care, to the Peace Corps. The pivotal concept of community was itself an infectious one, influential not only in mental health care but also in the design of contemporary antipoverty measures. Scholarly works highlight the part played by a coalition of reformist officials, liberal politicians, and mental health activists in moving community mental health legislation through the decision-making process (Foley 1975; Connery et al. 1968). More detailed background analysis relates this elite action to a historical context of shifting social understandings of the problem of mental illness and its treatment (Rochefort 1984).

A second school of thought looks beyond these auspicious beginnings of deinstitutionalization to some of its worst consequences, including inadequate follow-up services for discharged patients and large-scale transfers to such settings as nursing and boarding homes. In line with a neo-Marxist view of the state, this perspective views deinstitutionalization as a movement concerned less with patient welfare than with easing the growing public fiscal strain of institutional care. Deinstitutionalization thus represents a new style of community-based social control made possible by the advent of modern federal income maintenance and health insurance programs (Scull 1984). Brown (1985) also describes the development of a new medical-industrial complex under which public funds sustain the operation and profits of proprietary facilities.

Some reconciliation between these divergent characterizations is possible by recognizing deinstitutionalization as a disjointed, nonlinear process in which there has been "loose coupling" of policies and results (Gronfein 1985a). Kiesler and Sibulkin (1987) portray this discrepancy in terms of a distinction between de jure and de facto mental health policy, the former being the prescriptions of enacted law, while the latter is "the net outcome of overall practices, whether the outcome is intended or not." Other authors similarly describe deinstitutionalization less in terms of the rational unfolding of an overarching plan than as a hastily conceived, poorly managed undertaking whose thrust has altered over time and across the levels of government that became involved (Mechanic 1989; Lerman 1985; Rochefort 1987). Thus, inadvertence as well as design must be weighed in a complete account of the deinstitutionalization movement (Gronfein 1985a).

Deinstitutionalization Trends

Deinstitutionalization has been the "single most important issue" of concern for those in the mental health sphere for the past three decades (Rich 1986). An empirical examination of changes in the role played by public hospitals is central to understanding this process. In addition to an overall pattern of systemic transformation, the data reveal important variations in how this movement developed over time and at the state and local levels. Moreover, far from stimulating the phaseout of all types of institutional care, deinstitutionalization practices within state and county mental hospitals actually are associated with the rise of a variety of nontraditional institutions that have acquired an increasingly significant role in the custody and care of the mentally ill.

The National Scene

The most dramatic—and most commonly cited—statistic used to describe the course of deinstitutionalization in the United States is the year-end count of resident patients in state and county mental hospitals. From their initial appearance during the 1800s until the mid-twentieth century, these facilities underwent tremendous growth. From the start of the 1930s to 1955 alone, inpatient totals swelled from 332,000 to 559,000 (U.S. Bureau of the Census 1975:84, table B:423-27). This latter date marks the unofficial onset of deinstitutionalization, followed as it was by consistent annual census declines that only now may be abating (see table 8.1). Total resident patients at the end of 1986 numbered 109,000, an 81 percent reduction from thirty-one years earlier (NIMH 1989).

Table 8.1.
Resident Patients, Inpatient Episodes, and Admissions,
State and County Mental Hospitals, 1950 to 1985

Year	Year End Resident Patients	Inpatient Episodes	Admissions
1950	512,501		152,286
1955	558,922	818,832	178,003
1960	535,540		234,791
1965	475,202	804,926	316,664
1970	337,619		384,511
1975	193,436	598,993	376,156
1980	132,164		b
1985	109,939	459,374[a]	b

Source: NIMH (1989); Morrissey (1989:318-19, table 13-2).
[a] Figure cited is based on 1983
[b] After 1975, NIMH stopped reporting admissions and began reporting patient additions.

A second measure of hospital activity, and one that portrays the deinstitutionalization phenomenon in less drastic terms, is inpatient episodes. Cumulated over all facilities in the nation, this statistic takes account of resident census at the year's beginning, plus admissions, readmissions, and returns from leave during the reporting year. Total inpatient care episodes for state and county mental hospitals fluctuated in the neighborhood of 800,000 from 1955 to 1965. Thereafter, it fell steadily, reaching a level of 459,000 in 1983, or 44 percent below the 1955 number of 819,000. Compared to changes in the inpatient census, then, the number of inpatient episodes in public mental hospitals dropped much less precipitously and not until a decade after the resident patients' decline had gotten underway. The reason for the discrepancy in these two trend lines is that admissions to state and county mental hospitals—one of the principal components in the episodes calculation—continued to increase throughout the 1950s, 1960s, and early 1970s, offsetting until 1965 the simultaneous census reductions (Kiesler and Sibulkin 1987; Witkin et al. 1987).

At the same time that other operational measures have fallen, the period of time most inpatients spend within state and mental hospitals has also shortened. Average length of stay went from 421 days in 1969 to 143 days in 1982 (Kiesler and Sibulkin 1987). Median length of stay, a better measure of typical hospital stays, since its value is less sensitive to the inclusion of a comparatively small number of long-term inpatients, declined as well—from about 41 days in 1970 to 23 days in 1980 (Manderscheid et al. 1985).

Despite a general diminution in their service responsibilities, state and county mental hospitals have remained relatively stable in number over recent decades. In 1986, there were 286 such institutions in the United States, 11 more than in 1955. Between the two points in time, the highest count occurred in 1973, at 334 hospitals (NIMH 1989). On the other hand, the size of these public facilities assessed in terms of average number of inpatient beds has dropped sharply, from 1,311 in 1970 to 467 in 1984. Considered in conjunction with the nation's population growth during this same period, the change is noteworthy. Beds per 100,000 civilian population went from 207.4 in 1970 to 56.1 in 1984 (Witkin et al. 1987).

The Uneven Pace of Deinstitutionalization

Longitudinal analysis shows that deinstitutionalization did not occur at a steady rate (Gronfein 1985a; Lerman 1982, 1985). Inpatient declines during the late 1950s and first half of the 1960s were modest, especially compared to those that followed in the late 1960s and 1970s (see figure 8.1). Broken into a series of five-year intervals, the data show an aggregate decrease of only 4.2 percent for 1955 to 1960, and 11.3 percent for 1960 to 1965. By contrast, the cumulative decreases for 1965 to 1970, 1970 to 1975, and 1975 to 1980 were 29 percent, 42.7 percent, and 31.7 percent, respectively (calculated from NIMH 1989). Of the total census reduction of approximately 449,000 that took place between 1955 and 1985, more than three-quarters occurred in the period 1965 to 1980.

The major impact on deinstitutionalization of the federal health insurance and income maintenance programs that were established or expanded in the late 1960s and early 1970s has already been noted. The

FIGURE 8.1

Total Population
as a Percentage of 1955 Base

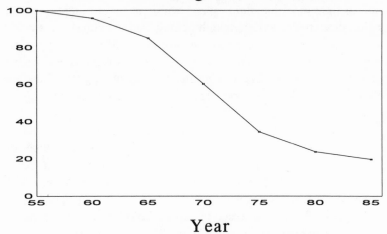

Year

Percentage Reduction
from Five Years Prior

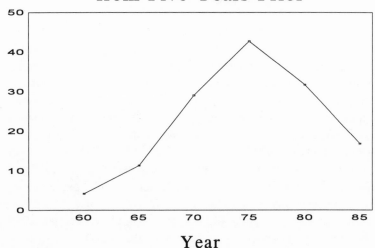

Year

Figure 8.1: Resident Patients in State and County Mental Hospitals: Total Population as a Percentage of 1955 Base and Percentage Reduction from Five Years Prior

above data further underscore the importance of these programs. Community mental health ideologies and even the availability of powerful tranquilizing drugs prior to 1965 failed on their own to drastically alter long-standing patterns of care. Only when these new ideas and treatments were joined by the financing of residential alternatives did the system respond on a large scale (Mechanic 1989).

Noting this unevenness in the historical development of deinstitutionalization, Morrissey (1982, 1989) describes two fundamentally different phases. The "benign" phase, which occurred between 1956 and 1965, consisted chiefly of "opening the back doors" of the state institutions to place new admissions and less impaired long-term residents in alternative settings. Many hospital treatment programs were also revitalized in this period. Following this was a "radical" phase from 1966 to 1975, which saw the "closing of the front doors" of these facilities. At a time when many states were experiencing economic hard times, hasty downsizing of residential populations and institutional capacity through patient diversions in addition to massive discharges provided a way of avoiding the expensive hospital improvement programs that new court and regulatory requirements often demanded. Community mental health and patient rights activists joined in support of this development.

Change at the Subnational Level

Corresponding to the lack of uniformity in deinstitutionalization over time is the striking variation among states. Table 8.2 provides information on the rates of public hospital depopulation across the states for two selected periods, 1967 to 1973 and 1973 to 1983. In both instances, values are widely dispersed—no single census reduction category contains as many as half of all states, and the difference between the highest- and lowest-ranking states in the later time frame exceeds 100 points (signifying that even in this, the heyday of deinstitutionalization, some states experienced a countertrend of hospital inpatient increases). Focusing on the 1956–65 and the 1966–75 periods, Gronfein (1985b) found the degree of interstate heterogeneity in deinstitutionalization to be greater during the earlier period. Rich (1986) similarly identifies several distinctive configurations for the pace and timing of state hospital inpatient declines in eighteen states between 1950 and 1978.

Table 8.2.
Percentage Reduction in Year-End Resident Patients by State Groupings,
1967 to 1973 and 1973 to 1983

Percentage Reduction	Number of States	
	1967-1973	1973-1983
0% or negative	0	3
1 - 20%	5	2
21 - 40%	23	11
41 - 60%	18	24
61 - 80%	5	10
81 - 100%	0	1
Mean reduction	38.8%	46.3%
Range	62.4	119.5
Standard deviation	15.1	23.2
Coefficient of variation	.39	.50

Source: Calculated from Taube (1975:15, table 4) and Greene et al. (1986:15, table 3).

Such variability is consistent with the idiosyncratic nature of individual state mental health systems, which developed for most of their histories free from the standardizing influence of a national mental health policy. A number of factors helped to shape differential state responses to the deinstitutionalization movement, including the starting condition of each state system in the late 1950s (e.g., the number of state hospitals and the size and composition of their populations); the relative strength of the political base of public mental institutions within the state; the fiscal structure of state mental health services, especially cost-sharing arrangements between state and community entities; the vigor and efficacy of the indigenous community mental health coalition, including its civil libertarian contingent; and the amount of economic strain faced by a given state with the stagflation of the 1970s (Morrissey 1982). Unfortunately, there are few detailed qualitative studies of individual state care systems in this period, making it difficult to trace the relative impacts of such determining features.

Table 8.3 shows state rates of deinstitutionalization between 1955 and 1973 (early) and between 1955 and 1986 (total). In the early phase, there was much variability, ranging from 14.7 percent in Nevada to 74.2 percent in California. The differential among states with the highest and lowest public hospital populations was large, with similar mean rates of deinstitutionalization among the large and small systems (57.7 percent versus 52.4 percent). By 1986, variation had been reduced, with rates of deinstitutionalization relative to the base year ranging from 60 percent to 90 percent. However, the difference in mean rates for the larger state systems for the period 1955–86 compared with those of smaller systems increased—a difference of 7.4 percent. Two of the small systems added to their inpatient populations between 1973 and 1986. These data reinforce the importance of considering specific conditions in force within states for understanding existing variation. The fact that all states depopulated mental hospitals to a significant extent reflects the common influences of ideology, technology, and federal entitlements and policies.

Role of CMHCs

Despite much rhetoric about their potential role, community mental health centers (CMHCs) did little to stimulate the depopulation of public hospitals (Torrey 1988; Mechanic 1989). In line with their comprehensive service mission, CMHCs have a heterogeneous clientele, with many users not seriously mentally ill. William Gronfein examined the change in numbers of patients in state and county mental hospitals in each state between 1973 and 1976 in relation to the number of inpatient CMHC beds, outpatient hours, day-care hours, and the percentage of catchment areas in each state with operating CMHCs (Gronfein 1985a). He found that greater CMHC activity was significantly associated with less deinstitutionalization, contrary to general beliefs. One explanation he suggests is that when CMHCs had greater resources, they were less motivated and less willing to become involved with public hospitals and chronic patients. In contrast, Medicaid payments for nursing home care were correlated (.82) with public mental hospital inpatient decline for the period 1970 to 1975, controlling for state population size. These data by themselves cannot support a causal argument, but they are consistent with the view that funding incentives under Medicaid facilitated inpatient reductions.

Table 8.3
Reduction in Public Mental Hospital Inpatients, 1955-1986, among States with Highest and Lowest Base Inpatient Populations in 1955

	States with Highest Number of Inpatients in 1955				
	Number of Inpatients			Percent decrease	
	1955	1973	1986	1955-73	1955-86
New York	94,175	44,963	22,033	52.3%	76.6%
Pennsylvania	39,834	19,023	6,779	52.2	83.0
Illinois	38,001	10,373	4,027	72.7	89.4
California	36,482	9,419	5,210	74.2	85.7
Ohio	28,116	12,903	4,307	54.1	84.7
Massachusetts	23,471	7,842	5,821	66.6	75.2
New Jersey	22,124	11,849	4,346	46.4	80.4
Michigan	21,249	7,563	4,891	64.4	77.0
Texas	16,553	9,937	4,090	40.0	75.3
Wisconsin	14,916	6,798	1,520	54.4	89.8
	States with Lowest Number of Inpatients in 1955				
	Number of Inpatients			Percent Decrease	
	1955	1973	1986	1955-73	1955-86
Nevada	416	355	136	14.7%	67.3%
Wyoming	639	304	254	52.4	60.3
New Mexico	1,059	450	219	57.5	79.3
Hawaii	1,232[a]	236	246	80.8	80.0
Idaho	1,247	270	188	78.3	84.9
Vermont	1,301	701	188	46.1	85.5
Utah	1,359	265	317	80.5	76.7
Delaware	1,414	1,169	516	17.3	63.5
South Dakota	1,595	942	419	40.9	73.7
Arizona	1,755	779	492	55.6	72.0

Sources: Figures for 1955 are from E.F. Torrey, *Nowhere to Go: The Tragic Odyssey of the Homeless Mentally Ill* (New York: Harper and Row, 1988), 219-20, appendix A. Figures for 1973 are from S. Greene et al., "State and County Mental Hospitals, United States, 1982-83 and 1983-84, with Trend Analysis from 1973-74 to 1983-84," *Statistical Note* 176 (National Institute of Mental Health, September 1986). Figures for 1986 are from M.J. Wilkin et al., "Specialty Mental Health System Characteristics," in *Mental Health, United States, 1990* (Washington, D.C.: U.S. Government Printing Office, 1990), 115-116, Table 1.21.
[a] Data for 1958 are from Hawaii State Mental Health Division.

Institutional Care

Deinstitutionalization did not produce a noninstitutional mental health system. Although the number of persons in state mental institutions was greatly reduced, the mental health system today still relies substantially on different forms of institutional care for the seriously mentally ill. Nursing homes have become a primary locus for the mentally ill; of the roughly 1.5 million nursing home residents in the United States today, estimates are that from 30 percent to more than 75 percent are mentally ill, depending on definitional criteria (Linn and Stein 1989). Private mental hospitals have also increased in size and number, in tandem with the down-scaling of state facilities.

The most dramatic growth, however, occurred in the general hospital sector, now the major provider of acute psychiatric inpatient care. Supported by the expansion of public and private mental health insurance benefits, admissions to specialized psychiatric services of general hospitals rose to 877,398 in 1988, an 84 percent increase since 1969 (Manderscheid 1991). Psychiatric admissions to general hospitals without psychiatric units brought the total to 1.56 million (Graves 1990). An estimated 300,000 to 400,000 mentally ill persons live in nontraditional institutions in the community—halfway houses, board-and-care homes, and other community residences (Segal and Kotler 1989).

State Hospitals

While the function of state mental hospitals has drastically changed over the past thirty-five years, such hospitals continue to provide a much-needed service within the overall mental health care system (Morrissey 1989). States have needed to reserve a supply of public beds for intermediate and long-term psychiatric care and for patients who are particularly difficult to manage in the general hospital sector due to their chronic conditions, legal status, or history of dangerous behavior. Consequently, even though state and county hospitals now account for a relatively small share of all inpatient mental health episodes each year, within the specialty mental health sector they are by far the largest provider of all inpatient days of mental health care, reflecting their clients' longer lengths-of-stay (table 8.4).

Table 8.4
Specialty Mental Health Sector Inpatient and Residential Treatment Days,
Number and Percent Distribution, Selected Years, 1969–1986

Type of organization	Thousands of Inpatient Days			
	1969	1975	1981	1986
All organizations	168,934	104,970	77,053	83,413
State and county mental hospitals	134,185	70,584	44,558	39,075
Private psychiatric hospitals	4,237	4,401	5,578	8,568
Nonfederal general hospitals with psychiatric services	6,500	8,349	10,727	12,570
Veterans medical centers	17,206	11,725	7,591	7,753
Federally funded CMHCs	1,924	3,718	-	-
Residential treatment centers for emotionally disturbed children	4,528	5,900	6,127	8,267
All other organizations	354	293	2,472	7,180
	Percent Distribution of Inpatient Days			
All organizations	100.0%	100.0%	100.0%	100.0%
State and county mental hospitals	79.4	67.2	57.8	46.8
Private psychiatric hospitals	2.5	4.2	7.2	10.3
Nonfederal general hospitals with psychiatric services	3.9	8.0	13.9	15.1
Veterans medical centers	10.2	11.2	9.9	9.3
Federally funded centers	1.1	3.5	-	-
Residential treatment centers for emotionally disturbed children	2.7	5.6	8.0	9.9
All other organizations	0.2	0.3	3.2	8.6

Source: National Institute of Mental Health, *Mental Health, United States, 1990* (Washington, DC: U.S. GPO, 1990), 34, table 1.5.
Note: In 1981, the federally funded community mental health centers (CMHCs) were combined with several other substance abuse programs to form the Alcohol, Drug Abuse, and Mental Health block grant. This led to a change in federal record keeping for the program.

Growth of the Mental Health System

Extraordinary growth of the mental health system coincided with deinstitutionalization. The number of patient care episodes in specialty mental health organizations went from 1.7 million in 1955 to 6.9 million in 1983 (Morrissey 1989) and to 7.9 million in 1988 (Manderscheid 1991). Community mental health centers, which did not exist before the mid-1960s, were treating as many as 3.3 million patients annually by the 1980s (Foley and Sharfstein 1983). Overall, Gerald Klerman has estimated a sixfold increase in the population's use of mental health services in the twenty-five years following 1955 (Klerman 1982).

This enlargement, which occurred alongside deinstitutionalization, complicates any evaluation of the program's impact. The need to accommodate new patient groups, many of whom never would have been candidates for state hospital admission in an earlier era, has been an independent force stimulating the shift to private and community-based services, irrespective of the deinstitutionalization movement.

Problems in the 1980s

Several factors combined in the 1980s to create a crisis in mental health services. Least anticipated within the mental health sector were the consequences of the changing demography of the American population, with large numbers of persons moving into age groups at high risk of mental illness. Schizophrenia and other major mental illnesses such as serious affective disorder and substance abuse commonly have their first occurrence in young adulthood. Given the demographic composition of the population, even if the incidence of disorder had remained unchanged, the prevalence of mental illness would have much increased.

Changing Demographics

Morton Kramer, former head of NIMH's Biometry Division, made extensive projections indicating increased service needs simply resulting from expected demographic changes, but these estimates elicited little interest and even less planning. For example, using census projections for the future U.S. population and specific age/ethnicity incidence rates for 1970 from the Monroe County, New York, Psychiatric Case Register, Kramer estimated incidence rates for schizophrenia between 1970 and 1985 (Kramer 1977). Assuming no change in specific age/ethnicity rates, he projected a growth in new cases of 21 percent, including an increase of 43 percent among nonwhites. These increases were expected to vary by age group, with projected increases of 56 percent among whites ages twenty-five to thirty-four, and 87 percent among nonwhites of that age. These increases were, of course, far in excess of expected percentage increases in the U.S. population. Kramer made comparable estimates for the period 1980–2005, projecting continued large increases in prevalence rates of serious mental disorders, especially among the nonwhite population (Kramer 1983).

There is no evidence of growth in the incidence of schizophrenia, but changes in household structure, the increase use of alcohol and drugs, and resistant attitudes to care among younger cohorts exposed to anti-mental health ideologies have seriously complicated the management of many of these patients. A variety of data sets suggest the possibility of an increased incidence of affective disorders among the young (Klerman and Weissman 1989). However, it remains unclear to what extent these findings can be explained by greater willingness among younger cohorts to recognize and report adverse psychological states and to seek care. Similarly, many mental health service programs care for elderly patients with Alzheimer's disease and other dementias—problems increasingly prevalent with the growth of the elderly population, particularly of those beyond age eighty who are more at risk. Based on growth in the population over age sixty-five, Kramer's estimates project a 44 percent increase in the number of persons with senile dementia between 1980 and 2005 (Kramer 1977).

Expansion of welfare policies in the mid-1960s facilitated deinstitutionalization, but the contraction of these policies in the 1980s, when most patients were already in the community and there was little access to public mental hospital beds, pushed the problem into the streets. Medicaid failed to keep pace with growth of the poor population, and eligibility, scope of services, and reimbursement to providers were restricted. Similarly, escalating disability costs led Congress to require states to review SSI and SSDI awards, a process intensified by the Reagan administration (Goldman and Gattozzi 1988). Between 1981 and 1983, half a million people lost benefits (Osterweis, Kleinman, and Mechanic 1987). Reviews of Social Security eligibility targeted younger recipients, disproportionately disenrolling mentally ill persons, who are on average much younger than those with chronic medical conditions. Several hundred thousand were reinstated on appeal, yet the loss of disability benefits created major difficulties in the mental health realm.

Housing

In the 1980s, housing opportunities shrank because of major cutbacks in federal housing programs, the gentrification of large city neighborhoods that housed the poor, and the loss of low-income housing. It was not until that decade, and the growing problem of homelessness, that mental health program administrators saw the need to develop appropriate housing for their client populations. By the middle 1980s, housing was seen as the single most critical issue faced by large city and state mental health authorities (Aiken, Somers, and Shore 1986).

The growth of homelessness, and the visibility of deranged persons on the streets, came to symbolize deinstitutionalization's failure as social policy. Public conceptions of the failures of deinstitutionalization are shaped by the media, which focus on the disorientation and pathetic situation of the homeless mentally ill in the nation's largest cities—a depiction not representative of the country as a whole. The problem of homelessness is commonly attributed to depopulation of public mental hospitals; in fact, the long-term patients discharged were predominantly white and middle-aged or elderly. Today's homeless are a heterogeneous population with disproportionate numbers of young black males and a significant minority of young women who have children but are unmarried or have disrupted marriages (Rossi and Wright 1989; Institute of Medicine 1988). While some discharged long-term patients undoubtedly became homeless, the two populations are quite different.

Numerous studies suggest that for many, homelessness is a temporary state reflecting the precarious situation of the poor during times of economic adversity or changing housing markets. While the poor who are housed possess many problems characteristic of the homeless population, the homeless poor have personal and social histories that make them particularly vulnerable during economic downturns, such as disrupted households, mental illness, substance abuse, arrest and imprisonment, weak family and personal networks, and poor coping skills.

Estimates of psychiatric problems among the homeless vary by the populations sampled and measurement criteria, but all studies report high morbidity and considerable prior contact with the mental health system, relative to the population as a whole. Incidents of acknowledged prior hospitalization vary from 1 to 33 percent among the homeless, in contrast to 3 to 7 percent among general adult community samples (Institute of

Medicine 1988). A study of the skid row homeless in Los Angeles using measures comparable to those of the NIMH Epidemiological Catchment Area Survey, which derived diagnostic judgments on the basis of interview responses, found that 60 percent of the homeless met criteria for mental illness or substance abuse disorder—about three times the general population rate (Institute of Medicine 1988). Peter Rossi, summarizing twenty-five studies of the homeless, estimates that 27 percent have a history of at least some mental hospital experience; a combination of seventeen studies suggests an average rate of chronic mental illness of 34 percent (Rossi and Wright 1989). These figures exceed those of other poor populations which are also vulnerable to psychiatric problems.

The homeless with substance abuse and mental health problems have numerous unmet service needs, but the vast majority do not require long-term hospitalization. Most are able to live in the community with appropriate supportive services and only occasionally require hospitalization, much like other patients with many other chronic diseases. A study of homeless persons in Baltimore found that substance abuse disorders were particularly high (75 percent for men and 38 percent for women), although major mental illnesses were also prevalent. The psychiatric investigators assessed 18 percent of the men and 15 percent of the women as needing short-term or intermediate inpatient psychiatric care, but only 1 percent were appropriate candidates for long-term hospitalization (Breakey et al. 1989). Furthermore, a study of men at initial entry into New York's municipal men's shelters indicated high levels of alcohol and drug abuse but fewer psychiatric problems. Only 17 percent were assessed as having a definite or probable history of psychosis (Susser, Struening, and Conover 1989). Those who had a history of homelessness prior to entering shelter care had more psychiatric problems. Thus, it appears that the seriously mentally ill are more likely than others to remain chronically homeless.

That the homelessness problem evades an easy solution is well illustrated by the fate of policy actions undertaken by the administration of former Mayor Ed Koch of New York City. Koch mounted an effort in the late 1980s to remove the mentally ill from the streets involuntarily to give them needed medical and psychiatric attention. In so doing, city officials loosely interpreted state commitment laws by applying the criterion of being in danger of causing serious harm to oneself or others "within the foreseeable future," rather than the standard legal test of "imminent danger." In addition to stimulating numerous legal challenges by those committed—including the celebrated case of Joyce Brown, who won release when the court blocked city doctors from administering medication to her against her will—the program led to overcrowded municipal hospital units, long patient lengths-of-stay, and attempts by the city to transfer large numbers of patients to state facilities. The essential reason for the backup was the unavailability of needed services, primarily housing and supervision, to support the return of patients to the community.

Homeless persons are often disadvantaged by poverty, alienation from social bonds, substance abuse, and serious mental and physical illnesses. They need services that are either in short supply or unavailable. Very few of these patients require long-term hospitalization, but many require decent housing and appropriate mental health and alcohol and drug abuse treatment and rehabilitation. Hospitals are a form of housing, but at a prohibitive price for those who do not need these specialized environments. The cost of public hospitalization in new York exceeds $100,000 per person each year.

Estimating the costs of hospital and community care relative to benefits involves a variety of difficult methodological issues on what measures to include, the time span to consider for analysis, and indicators of costs and benefits (Rubin 1990). Burton Weisbrod and colleagues did one of the most systematic studies, comparing the experience of experimental and control groups in the Wisconsin Program in Assertive Community Treatment (PACT) (Weisbrod, Test, and Stein 1980). They found that this intensive program cost somewhat more per patient than traditional care ($8,093 versus $7,269) but resulted in a somewhat superior cost/benefit outcome. The experimental program studied, however, was extremely service-intensive. Most cost/benefit comparisons find alternatives to mental hospitals far less costly, but these analyses typically lack the comprehensiveness and sophistication of the PACT evaluation (Kiesler and Sibulkin 1987). Hospital care, however, has become highly expensive in most acute general hospitals and in many state systems. In most instances, very intensive outpatient services and related social and welfare services can be provided at lower cost, motivating the development of intensive case management programs. The challenge is to focus services on patients who will be high users of future inpatient care, a task that can be difficult (Weissert 1985).

Deinstitutionalization and Other Problem Populations

Over the past few decades deinstitutionalization has emerged as a principal theme of policy and practice in several other human service areas as well, including developmental disability, physical disability, and corrections (DeJong 1979; Lerman 1982, 1985; Scull 1984). Dimensions of this movement are reflected in such measures as a decline in the rate of institutionalization in state mental retardation facilities (from 97.7 per 100,000 in 1965 to 46.8 per 100,000 in 1985) (U.S. Bureau of the Census 1987), reduced use of public training schools for delinquents (whose rate of institutionalization dropped from 98 to 69 per 100,000 youths over 1970–77) (Lerman 1985), and the increasing percentage of releases on parole from state prisons in the 1960s and 1970s (attaining a level as high as 70 percent) (Sykes 1978). More recently, there has also been increasing use of supervised home release for prisoners.

Several key parallels can be drawn between developments within these other deinstitutionalizing areas and mental health (DeJong 1979; Sykes 1978; Lerman 1982, 1985; Rothman 1980; Scheerenberger 1983; Scull 1984; Tyor and Bell 1984). As a frequent scenario, the deinstitutionalization impulse emanated from a combination of sources—ideological, judicial, and economic. In part, there was intellectual cross-fertilization from mental health to these other fields, but each field also gave birth to its own concepts. Typically, court orders insisted on improved institutional conditions, and availability of increased federal funding for new services also shaped alternatives. Growth of nontraditional institutional forms (halfway houses, foster homes, group homes, treatment centers, etc.) developed in all sectors. And in every case, deinstitutionalization eventually stimulated public debate over the method and impacts of program implementation. But important differences exist between these other human service systems and mental health. No other area experienced the scope of deinstitutionalization characteristic of the mental health sector. Institutional-noninstitutional patterns within these respective systems also vary. Whereas new service modalities in mental health developed mostly parallel to traditional institutions and as an alternative, in mental retardation many new residential care facilities are physically a part of the state institution (Lerman 1985). Similarly, expanded community programs in criminal justice, unlike mental health, operate in tandem with a sharply increasing institutional population and a movement to construct additional prison facilities (Scull 1984; *New York Times* 17 May 1987).

Deinstitutionalization in Perspective

Deinstitutionalization arose from complex interacting social forces, was implemented with startling rapidity, and is now beset by political and professional controversy. Such circumstances are conducive to misperception and misunderstanding. Clearly, state and county mental hospitals no longer occupy the preeminent position they once did within the U.S. mental health system. By the same token, however, one should not neglect the significant place that these institutions maintain in contemporary mental health services. By a wide margin, state hospitals remain the foremost provider of total inpatient days of psychiatric care (Kiesler and Sibulkin 1987), and they care for many of the most difficult, troubled, and violent patients. These institutions also continue to house a sizable number of long-term patients—according to one estimate, nearly 20 percent of their patient population at any point has been hospitalized for twenty years or more (Morrissey 1989). State hospitals are reported to absorb nearly two-thirds of the expenditures of state mental health agencies (Lutterman et al. 1987), although these figures may be exaggerated by the way such data are collected—hospital outreach and community care programs are reported as part of hospital expenditures and not as a contribution to community care.

Extraordinary growth in the mental health sector as a whole coincided with the deinstitutionalization movement, and it is perhaps this conjunction of historical occurrences that induces premature reports of the death of the public mental hospital. An important change from inpatient to outpatient care underlay this increase: in 1955, the distribution of episodes favored inpatient care by a 3.42:1 ratio; in 1983, the ratio was 2.69:1 in favor of outpatient care (Morrissey 1989:318–19, table 13–2; Thompson, Bass, and Witkin 1982). With more persons being treated for mental illness, the probability of a typical patient having contact with state and county mental hospitals has been much lowered (Morrissey 1989). Most patients now being treated by community agencies and alternative institutional facilities would not have been in public mental health systems in prior decades. This overall growth of the mental health sector has played a major part in the transformation of the role of state and county mental hospitals (Kiesler and Sibulkin 1987), which have increasingly become the system of last resort for the uninsured, the treatment resistant, and those who are most difficult to relocate to other settings.

The growth of health insurance covering mental health benefits, concurrent with deinstitutionalization, helped transform mental health care. The most significant single change was the development of the general community hospital as the major site for acute psychiatric inpatient care. Many general hospitals developed specialized psychiatric units. Medicaid became a major source of payment for inpatient psychiatric care in general hospitals for many chronic patients, contributing to a pattern of episodic hospital care characterized by short lengths of stay with little community follow-up (Mechanic 1989).

As care for the most severely mentally ill patients shifted from public institutions to community care settings, the functions traditionally associated with public mental hospitals remained but were now more dispersed among varying community agencies and different levels of government. Severely disabled patients still required medical and psychiatric care, housing, psychosocial and educational services, a program of activities, assistance in attaining welfare benefits, and supervision of their medication and daily routines. The strategic task of integrating these functions outside of institutions is a formidable one, and there is persistent evidence of failure in meeting these needs in even the most rudimentary ways (Torrey 1988; Mechanic 1989).

A Note on Cross-National Experience

Even in the United States deinstitutionalization proceeded differentially among the states, depending on the structure of their mental health systems, social and economic conditions, the power base of interested constituencies, and the strength of the mental health reform movement. Comparative analysis is extremely difficult with nations varying greatly in their economic and political systems and in the structure of their health care and welfare services. Some analysts examine deinstitutionalization in the context of the rise of the welfare state and the way "in which group interests were aggregated, represented and mediated," and its specific urban manifestations (Dear and Wolch 1987). However, few studies garner data from localities in more than one or two countries.

Information and new technical approaches diffuse rapidly throughout the world, and thus, ideas about deinstitutionalization and the value of neuroleptic drugs were widely available in the developed countries by the late 1950s. Moreover, experience in community living for the mentally impaired has long existed as in Gheel (Belgium) and other communities. In contrast, ideologies, leadership, political participation, social control, and the organization of health and welfare are not only specific to nation, but also to locality. In England, a source of many of the social psychiatric ideas about community care, the population of mental hospitals began to fall around 1954 with the introduction of reserpine and chlorpromazine, ideas about therapeutic communities, and change in administrative practices (Brown et al. 1966; Wing and Brown 1970). Despite much experimentation with alternatives and rehabilitation approaches, deinstitutionalization in Britain never developed the momentum seen in the United States. Many reasons may account for the contrast, including the fact that British psychiatry is a hospital-based consulting specialty, the focus of interest in Britain on therapeutic hospital alternatives, a cultural environment supporting incremental change, and a different social history in the management of the impaired elderly.

Canada followed a similar course to the United States, although deinstitutionalization occurred later and to a smaller extent. In Ontario, for example, patients in provincial asylums increased until 1960 to a peak of almost 19,507 but by 1976 was 5,030 (Dear and Wolch 1987). Deinstitutionalization in Australia has accelerated in recent years, influenced by American programs (Hoult 1987).

Despite these commonalities, deinstitutionalization has not been universal. In much of Europe, where a medically oriented, hospital-based psychiatry is dominant, the treatment of serious mental illness remains substantially centered in hospitals. In Austria, for example, there is extremely strong resistance to community-based care and little deinstitutionalization. In Japan, private psychiatric hospitals are growing rapidly and are replacing informal sources of care. Deinstitutionalization must be seen in relation to a nation's values and in the historical context of its political, economic, social, and health and welfare institutions.

In recent years much attention has focused on deinstitutionalization in Italy, and particularly in Trieste, which closed its mental hospital. This movement, based on the ideology of Franco Basaglia, a Venetian psychiatrist, viewed hospitalization as psychiatric repression and deinstitutionalization as one element of a class struggle. As in the United States in the 1960s, hospitalization is viewed as a cause of illness and disability. The dilemmas of mental illness are explained in the light of struggles among interests over power and control of social institutions (Lovell 1985). Good data are difficult to obtain, and there is much controversy and conflicting views about the changes that have spread throughout Italy. There is indication of significant transfer of patients to other institutions, no longer called hospitals. As in the United States, the evaluation of the consequences of change depend very much on appraisals of local situations in a context of large variability.

Impact of Deinstitutionalization and Future Needs

The long-term care patients who had been resident in mental hospitals prior to deinstitutionalization, if still surviving, are now relatively elderly and are not a major focus of the controversy that rages around the issue of deinstitutionalization. Indeed, long-term studies of the course of schizophrenia in the United States and abroad demonstrate persuasively that with time the most severe symptoms abate and schizophrenic patients can make reasonable adjustments to the community (Harding et al. 1987a, 1987b; Bleuler 1978; Ciompi 1980). Older U.S. patients released from mental hospitals were relocated in nursing homes, sheltered care facilities, and families. Some were demented patients who had been kept in mental hospitals because of a lack of alternative institutional settings. Others were elderly patients whose psychotic symptoms had substantially abated but who retained social disabilities due to their long confinements.

The deinstitutionalization debate confuses this now aged population which was relocated from public hospitals to other settings during the decades of rapid deinstitutionalization, with new cohorts of seriously mentally ill patients who are now part of an entirely different system of care (Mechanic 1987). It is this younger population of patients with psychoses and personality disorders, socialized in different cultural and treatment contexts, who are often difficult to manage and who frighten the community. These younger patients often resist the idea that they are mentally ill, are uncooperative with treatment, abuse alcohol and drugs, and generally live an unconventional style of life (Schwartz and Goldfinger 1981; Sheets, Prevost, and Reihmank 1982; Pepper and

Ryglewicz 1982). Much of the debate, however it is framed, really focuses on this new and growing population of severely mentally ill youth and young adults. The problem is exacerbated by demographic trends that result in large subgroups in the population at ages of high risk for occurrence of schizophrenia and substance abuse (Mechanic 1987).

In the United States, the problems have also become more visible and acute with the contraction of public programs during the 1980s. Recall that the large waves of deinstitutionalization occurred with the expansion of social welfare activities in the late 1960s and 1970s, particularly Medicaid, SSI and SSDI, housing programs, and food stamps. These programs provided the subsistence base essential for relocating patients to the community. This subsistence base was not maintained relative to the growing numbers of seriously mentally ill persons, and in many instances it substantially shrank. The cutbacks in social programs particularly affected the seriously mentally ill. The mentally ill have been particularly vulnerable because they typically lack bureaucratic skills to gain eligibility to social programs, and administrators who run many welfare programs have little appreciation of their special needs. In addition, the mentally ill suffer considerable stigma and discrimination relative to other eligible competing groups such as the poor elderly. In recent years, mental health programs have become more aggressive in helping the mentally ill attain eligibility for Medicaid, SSI, and housing benefits, but in an environment of shrinking resources.

Strategies for Integrating Public Mental Health Services

Almost every observer notes models of public mental health services that are more successful than conventional treatment, but bemoans that such models are not widely adopted. The reasons posited for the lack of dissemination usually include dispersion of responsibility and authority, the lack of professional incentives, perverse financial inducements, the bureaucratization of care, the influence of entrenched interest groups, legal obstacles, and a lack of interest among influential public officials. These portrayals contain much truth, but they provide no clear direction for the implementation of improved systems of care.

Explanations for the failures of mental health services are almost interchangeable with those offered for the array of human services problems that affect the disadvantaged. These analyses fault the broader social dynamics of our federal system in which responsibilities and authority are dispersed across executive, legislative, and judicial sectors, among a range of bureaucratic agencies, and different levels of government. Thus a common complaint is the massive difficulties faced in integration and coordination at the service level.

It would be unduly optimistic to assume that American political traditions will be modified to accommodate the need to solve problems of fragmentation of public mental health services. Practical solutions must be developed within existing political structures.

Frameworks of Care

Adequate financing of mental health care, and insurance coverage of mental health services, are essential enabling factors for adequate public mental health care, but in addition, there must be viable frameworks for organizing the effective delivery of services. Many localities have substantial resources but use them inefficiently; thus the relationship between per capita expenditures of public mental health resources and the quality of public mental health services is modest (Torrey, Erdman, and Wolfe 1990). Mental health authorities, of course, work with different levels of complexity; it is easier to develop integrated systems of care in small states like Maine, New Hampshire, and Vermont than in large urban areas where mental health planning is complicated by population density; racial and ethnic heterogeneity; a lack of affordable housing; high rates of AIDS, crime, and other pathologies; and intense special interest politics.

There are at least four generic approaches to building a viable public mental health system: developing assertive community treatment systems; capitating mental health care; building strong local mental health authorities; and developing supportive reimbursement structures.

Each of these strategies typically is implemented in isolation, but developing a strong thrust for change will require a more integrated approach. It is essential that mental health care providers understand clearly how best to meet clinical and psychosocial needs, but the stability and effectiveness of public mental health services also depend on the financial and organizational frameworks that underlie clinical efforts.

Providing Assertive Community Treatment

Bringing together the services that mental patients need in the community requires a strong organizational capacity, a clear focus of longitudinal responsibility, and the ability to guide available funds. Several controlled clinical trials and other studies consistently show that most organized alternatives to mental hospital care have outcomes as good as or better than traditional inpatient treatment and aftercare (Kiesler and Sibulkin 1987, Stein and Test 1985). However, most of the programs, and the studies evaluating them, have been carried out in geographic areas of modest size, which means that the challenges of coordination are not as formidable as in large cities. Even so, the sociopolitical contexts of the alternative programs are not atypical of areas in which large populations of mentally ill persons reside.

These studies show that the severely mentally ill treated in aggressively organized programs of care can be successfully retained in the community. Some studies, such as those based on the Program for Assertive Community Treatment (PACT) in Dane County, Wisconsin, also found that patients in those programs function better and report a higher quality of life than patients receiving more conventional hospital and outpatient care, but that care must be sustained over time to maintain favorable results (Stein and Test 1980; Davis, Pasamanick, and Dinitz 1974). Studies on related programs also find significantly reduced inpatient care but have not reported comparable reductions of symptoms and improved functioning (Olfson 1990).

Stein, one of the originators of the Dane County model, has argued that it is inappropriate to treat different assertive community treatments as comparable. Describing the Dane County model as it is operating today, he advocates a system that uses a multidisciplinary, assertive, continuous care team that "serves as a fixed point of responsibility for a designated group of patients with severe and persistent mental illness and is concerned with all aspects of their lives that influence their functioning." (Stein 1990) These teams, working with patients in homes, neighborhoods, and work places, provide varying intensities of service, depending on patient need, and are available on a twenty-four-hour basis. Teams also work with community members, act as gatekeepers to inpatient care, and help coordinate care when patients are hospitalized.

We still know relatively little about which subcomponents of the Dane County model are most important for improved outcomes. The model is a complex system of interventions that is unlikely to be adopted in its totality in other sociopolitical, financial, and clinical environments. To the extent that the system must be translated as a whole, it will be more difficult to disseminate it widely. It remains unclear whether variations in outcome that have been found when the model is only partly replicated are due solely to treatment differences or to other factors such as varying patient populations, medication compliance, and quality of administrative and clinical management. To assess the generalizability of various elements of the Dane County model, it would be necessary to conduct a multisite study in differing geographic contexts using a standard protocol.

The Dane County approach has been adopted more widely than most mental health service innovations, but the model and its variations, even after two decades, serve relatively few patients. Stein and his colleagues (Stein and Ganser 1983; Stein 1989) emphasize the importance of Wisconsin's system of mental health financing, in which the state gives the counties a global budget that allows them to trade outpatient for inpatient care. It remains unclear, however, why so few of Wisconsin's fifty-five mental health boards have developed a system equal to Dane County's, and why some county systems continue to operate as hospital-oriented systems. Nor is it clear why other states with comparable financing incentives vary so greatly in the kinds of systems that evolve.

Stein (1989) has emphasized the importance of transitional funds in converting from a hospital- to a community-based system. He also argues that community-based systems, unlike many medical care innovations, have to overcome a variety of barriers. Such innovations typically are developed in public settings and conflict with dominant traditions, philosophies, and practices in the field. They require changes in professional roles and restructuring of hierarchical status systems. Also, the major training programs for the mental health professions reinforce traditional patterns of practice.

Although Stein offers a plausible explanation for the sluggishness of the diffusion of the Dane County model, his analysis does not make clear how these barriers can be overcome. The variations among sociopolitical contexts and professional settings may require compromises when adopting the basic model, but if the compromises yield less promising results, the incentive to take the trouble diminishes. This situation suggests, even more forcefully, the importance of identifying the most therapeutic components of such complex programs. Early work by Rosenfield on patients' overall quality of life, based on a club model used elsewhere, suggests the importance of an empowerment philosophy and the structuring of patients' activities, particularly on nights and weekends (Rosenfield 1992).

Capitating Mental Health Care

The Wisconsin Financing System, Stein (1989) argues, provides an incentive for preventing unnecessary hospital care because the community care team understands that if they spend too much money on inpatient treatment, little funding will remain to support their jobs in the community. Such an incentive may exist once a system of community care is in place and employees develop a stake in it, but Wisconsin's type of financing does not necessarily push any local system of care in this direction.

Capitation funding offers more powerful incentives to move the service delivery system in new directions (Mechanic and Aiken 1989). Capitation has three specific features: all defined services for a specified time period are provided through an agreed-on prepayment; payment is tied to the care of a particular patient; and the provider, in accepting the capitation, agrees to be at risk for costs exceeding the capitation amount. Thus, the provider has an incentive to manage carefully, and to avoid unnecessary expensive treatment such as inpatient care.

Such incentives, of course, always involve some risks of the withholding of necessary care (Schlesinger 1989). Wisconsin's system of financing allows managed care but, unlike capitation, does not entail financial risk for providers unless they develop a stake in alternative systems of care. Capitation, by tying care to particular patients, could also be a powerful device for redirecting care to less attractive patients who often are rejected by providers. Capitation payments can be adjusted to the needs and qualities of varying types of patients.

Capitation for seriously ill mental patients is seen as a way to bring fragmented funding streams together, providing resources to develop new services. Such systems of care, however, are complex endeavors, and few administrators of mental health systems have the technical expertise or professional self-confidence to negotiate the necessary agreements, calculate the appropriate capitation allowances, or to work out complicated arrangements for sharing risk. Realizing the potential benefits of capitation depends on bringing Medicaid funding into the system, but working out the necessary state and federal arrangements is a formidable task. These factors explain the gap between interest in capitation and implementation of a capitation system.

A partial capitation system has been used successfully by the state of Rhode Island to close some hospital units (Mauch 1989). Long-term patients were returned to the community, and capitation financing was provided as an additional incentive to separately funded community mental health centers to focus more attention on these usually neglected patients. Unlike the situation in full capitation systems, the centers were never put at risk of loss of budget if they managed care inefficiently.

The most ambitious capitation effort yet attempted is in Rochester, New York, where, after many years of development, a nonprofit voluntary corportation called Integrated Mental Health, Inc., was established to administer a capitation program for seriously mentally ill patients in Monroe and Livingston counties (Babigian and Marshall 1989). Early results indicate that clinical outcomes comparable to those from conventional care can be achieved at much lower cost (Babigian 1990). As in other capitation programs, the focus has been on patients recently treated as inpatients in a state psychiatric facility, although the program also includes nonhospitalized mentally ill persons.

Capitation approaches are intuitively appealing, particularly as an opportunity for building systems. If enough patients are included, the resource fund for developing new services could be substantial. Also, capitation provides a clear incentive for giving attention to targeted patients. But the complexity of capitation systems, the technical knowledge required, and the high start-up costs pose formidable barriers to widespread adoption. The possibilities for using capitation increase as stronger mental health authorities develop.

Developing Local Mental Health Authorities

In most localities, no single organization, either in government or the nonprofit sector, takes the responsibility or has the authority to guarantee the range of services the mentally ill need. A key deficiency is that few mental health agencies are able to consolidate the variety of funding streams, which limits their ability to set priorities and allocate funds for them.

The effectiveness of administrative arrangements depends on the political culture of the locality and on the extent to which these arrangements are consistent with the local legal framework, traditions, and political alignments. State and local governments administer mental health services in varied ways. One strategy has been to encourage the development of central authorities that can consolidate administrative, fiscal, and clinical responsibility for care; the Robert Wood Johnson Foundation has funded a demonstration program in nine large cities for the development of such authorities to plan and provide services to chronic mentally ill persons (Aiken, Somers, and Shore 1986).

Consolidating political authority is no easy matter, nor is it clear that the entities that evolve would necessarily improve the integration of services and quality of care. Yet theoretically it seems reasonable to expect that if administrative entities have greater capability to manage care within a consolidated budget, services will improve. An extensive evaluation of the nine-city demonstration program is in process, and we are likely to learn a great deal about the potentialities and difficulties of the task (Goldman, Lehman et al. 1990).

The development of a new administrative authority is a long-term task. In the nine cities in the demonstration program, central mental health authorities have not evolved as quickly or operated as comprehensively as many people anticipated (Goldman, Morrissey et al. 1990). Even local participants underestimated the organizational and political barriers to centralizing control, particularly the difficulty of gaining increased control over state hospital funding. The program is showing that individual participants can agree on the importance of central control and the need to integrate, but that organizational entities, professional groups, and public administrators are not particularly ready to yield their influence to other groups. The endorsements of governors, mayors, and other high public officials were sought by the foundation in selecting the cities for the demonstration program, but endorsements go only so far when power and control are at stake.

Some significant gains may result from the development of more influential mental health authorities, but these efforts alone will not be a panacea. A key problem all authorities face is how to effectively use reimbursement incentives to elicit the desired services.

Structuring Reimbursement

Reimbursement is often said to be the force that drives the service delivery system. In recent years much effort has been devoted to designing reimbursement approaches that encourage efficient use of resources, such as the Medicare Prospective Payment System (Russell 1989), but reimbursement can also be designed to focus attention on neglected populations or to change patterns of service (Frank and Lave 1985, 1989; Siegel et al. 1986).

Mental health systems increasingly depend on psychiatric units in general hospitals to be the first line of response in dealing with serious mental illness. Medicaid is the primary source of payment for about one-quarter of all such psychiatric admissions nationally. In New York State, approximately 35 to 40 percent of psychiatric admissions to specialized units in general hospitals are covered by Medicaid, giving the state system a large stake in patterns of care in these hospitals. Beginning in October 1989, under a system called the Consolidated Inpatient and Outpatient Psychiatric Rate Methodology, New York State designed a series of financial incentives for general hospitals with specialized psychiatric units to encourage them to treat more people with serious and persistent mental illness and to link them with outpatient programs after discharge (Rutgers Center for Research on the Organization and Financing of Care for the Severely Mentally Ill 1991). Under the program, twenty-seven of the state's municipal and general hospitals with psychiatric units were reimbursed under the new rates during the first year, with the rates to be phased in at all such hospitals over four years.

Many of New York's problems in providing general psychiatric care are common to much of the nation. Many patients with serious and persistent mental illness have difficulty getting access to inpatient care. When they are admitted, their length of stay may be so short that they cannot receive a serious evaluation, or so long that it blocks access to beds needed by other patients. Despite the high costs of inpatient care, readmission rates are high. Discharge planning is often inadequate, and patients are often not linked with necessary aftercare. In New York, for example, only 30 percent of Medicaid patients discharged from inpatient care are linked to outpatient clinic services within a month, and only 40 percent within a year. The intensity of outpatient services is too low in relation to patient need. Patients are often lost in the community after hospital discharge and not uncommonly become homeless.

In redesigning its reimbursement system for psychiatric care, New York State sought to use financial incentives to achieve several objectives: to focus more attention on the most neglected populations—persistently mentally ill patients and children; to increase the overall inpatient capacity of the system without adding expensive new beds; to encourage improved discharge planning and early outpatient linkage; to increase the intensity of outpatient aftercare for the most persistently mentally ill patients and reduce repeated admissions; and to generally improve coordination between the inpatient and outpatient systems of care. Unlike many reimbursement approaches, this new methodology is not intended to contain costs. However, proponents believe that a more responsive system of community care will make it possible to decrease the number of public beds and thus reduce public mental hospital expenditures in the long run.

The experience, thus far, suggests that the new reimbursement methodology has fallen below expectations and has not contributed a great deal to achieving the goals envisioned. The reimbursement methodology was introduced during a period of considerable economic problems and organizational disarray, during which large cuts in reimbursement and services were implemented, and hospitals were functioning in a turbulent environment. It was not clear that the new incentives had much impact relative to other changes affecting the system. Nor was it clear that the incentives were large enough to change behavior or that those who had to implement the necessary changes saw any direct relationship between their behavior and the rewards accruing to their programs. Further, it was unclear that any increased reimbursement paid to the hospital would necessarily be awarded to the psychiatric unit, thus weakening motives to change.

The lesson to be learned is that while reimbursement is a powerful lever, it must be calibrated to the magnitude of the task envisioned. It is not clear that the incentives were large enough at the margins to motivate hospitals to take more of the designated clients. Moreover, there should be a direct link between the incentive payments and the reinforcement of behavior. Even if mental health professionals believed that the incentive payments would return to the psychiatric unit, the complicated way in which the reimbursement incentives were paid weakened a clear link between behavior and reward.

Despite this particular experience, it is evident that reimbursement is one of the key levers available to alter the existing configuration of services to a more desirable one. Such reimbursement strategies, however, are directed at changing behavior reflecting particular values, goals and cultures. Thus, such strategies must be carefully devised and communicated, and the incentives must be strong enough and clearly perceived to counteract other forces affecting behavior.

Conjoint Strategies

Each of the four generic strategies—assertive community treatment, capitation, local mental health authorities, and new reimbursement structures—addresses somewhat different system needs. Achieving the potential of these approaches depends on the ability to combine them in a mutually reinforcing way. Many localities are now developing assertive community treatment and other case management modalities, but without a coherent, structured system of care and financial incentives that reinforce it, these approaches are fragile. Capitation, by itself, creates incentives for managed care and resource development. But it does not ensure optimal clinical decision making and may, in the absence of clear clinical direction or quality assurance mechanisms, erect deterrents to needed care. Joining capitation to an assertive care program creates a potential for benefiting from the special features of the funding arrangement while maintaining a clear focus on clinical priorities.

Strong mental health authorities of the kind envisioned by the Robert Wood Johnson project provide a broader framework for organizing assertive community treatment while developing the financial and administrative capacity to plan, develop, and manage capitation. Such models as Rochester's Integrated Mental Health, Inc. have multiple roles in planning, resource development, financial administration (as in the Rochester capitation plan), and the development of a sophisticated management information system.

The fate of all the above endeavors depends on the level of financing of mental health care and the incentives that shape professional and institutional behavior. Reimbursement arrangements can be strong stimuli for increasing underdeveloped services such as psychosocial rehabilitation (now allowable under Medicaid) or for directing attention to neglected groups of patients. Many needed modalities, such as housing and structured day, evening, and weekend programs, depend on conditions beyond favorable systems of reimbursement. But a reimbursement strategy that is consistent with, and reinforces, major priorities such as new residential options and assertive case management, establishes the necessary conditions for a strong and stable system. Rarely do we give enough attention to bringing compatible strategies together, although such an enterprise provides an important opportunity for significant change.

There is no quick fix for the problems that plague public mental health systems. The problems are deeply entrenched and difficult to solve. Many public officials are concerned that investments in mental health will not yield significant visible benefits that justify taking political risks. However, a conjoint strategy that establishes responsible and accountable community entities that are sensitive to efficient financial approaches and responsive to clinical issues offers significant potential. Implementation will require active and sustained support from mental health advocates.

Challenges of Deinstitutionalization as Public Policy

The notion of returning to a state hospital-centered mental health system would be unrealistic today, even if such a course was seen as desirable. Thirty-five years of deinstitutionalization and growth of a broad range of services have resulted in a decentralized, pluralistic mental health sector funded by a diversity of public and private programs. Thus, a monolithic hospital-based system is an impractical model from both an organizational and political standpoint. Especially in this era of government deficits, it would be prohibitively expensive to upgrade and expand hospital facilities to the point at which they could provide a decent living environment and continuous appropriate treatment to large numbers of patients. A well-planned, treatment-oriented, hospital-based system is not inconceivable, but without substantial reinvestment, state mental hospitals would quickly degenerate into the human warehouses of the past. Moreover, a policy of long-term institutionalization is inconsistent with the principle of care in the least restrictive setting that now stands as accepted legal doctrine in our society and is the conditioned expectation of persons who receive mental health services. Finally, the idea of a hospital-based system is inconsistent with a large body of research showing that alternatives to hospitalization improve function and quality of life relative to hospital-based care (Kiesler and Sibulkin 1987).

The impulse for reinstitutionalization reflects a long-standing tendency within the mental health field toward vacillation between hospital and community alternatives (Rochefort 1988). These debates typically neglect the complex nature and variety of mental disorders and the full spectrum of service programs required (Grob 1987b). The present challenge of deinstitutionalization as public policy is to avoid this cyclical trend by ensuring that community and hospital sectors come to play complementary roles in an integrated system, providing patients with care suited to their distinctive needs and capabilities. Necessary reforms in mental health financing and service delivery have already been described. We turn to examining some of the larger social policy issues.

Deinstitutionalization is one of a group of social initiatives of the 1960s that began with great expectations but resulted in a neoconservative backlash against government interventionism. In the case of many of these initiatives, including deinstitutionalization, a distorted public image has taken hold that exaggerates the dimensions of failure while ignoring positive accomplishments (Schwarz 1988). Even in a more balanced assessment, however, the reality of disappointing performance is plain and underscores the difficulty of translating reformist policy design into effective programmatic action. It is a subject that has come to be known in the policy sciences literature as the "implementation problem" (Bardach 1977; Williams 1980).

Implementation difficulties have undermined the deinstitutionalization effort from its inception and are evident in such basic disjunctions as the neglected relationship between community mental health centers and state hospitals. Coordination processes of this nature, like those essential to the creation of a comprehensive sociomedical support system for chronically mentally ill persons in the community, represent the classic implementation challenge. They require the long-term cooperation of multiple service bureaucracies and levels of government. What makes the task so hard—and what promises to test case management, special mental health authorities, and other current approaches in the mental health system—are overlapping issues of territoriality, resource supply, technical capability, and conflicting organizational objectives and styles (Dill and Rochefort 1989). In attempting to overcome these obstacles, mental health professionals and administrators confront the powerful force of tradition and an American human services apparatus built around the concept of dispersed responsibility.

Uncertainty about control and accountability in mental health care at the level of service delivery is matched by persistent ambivalence on these questions within government as a whole. Here, again, problems experienced by the mental health sphere reflect broader social policy dynamics of our federal political order.

The provision of public mental health services began as a local responsibility in the colonial era. With the spread of public mental hospitals in the 1800s, the task then shifted to the states. The Community Mental Health Centers Act of 1963 staked out a national interest in mental health care, one consciously designed to bypass the state role, which was viewed as too tradition-bound for the necessary reforms. Roughly thirty years later, the Reagan administration's Alcohol, Drug Abuse, and Mental Health block grant decentralized administrative responsibility for this community mental health program to state officials. At the same time, however, the national government continues to seek to provide leadership—and a set of common priorities—in mental health policy through its ongoing work to bring psychiatric services in general hospitals into Medicare's prospective payment system, and through legislation to provide funding for such purposes as state mental health planning (Public Law 99-660) and services for the homeless mentally ill (Public Law 100-77) (Levine and Haggard 1989). It also exerts a massive indirect influence on mental health policy through general entitlement programs and the administrative regulations that govern these. A tangled, unresolved intergovernmental relationship results that makes it exceedingly difficult to develop rational or even coherent policy.

The low standing of mental health issues on the national social agenda poses another impediment to needed improvement of the mental health system. Except for brief interludes in American history, the mentally ill have not captured the serious attention of elected officials, who generally have little interest or knowledge relating to mental illness. The rule, instead, has been neglect and a failure to appreciate the scope, severity, and degree of dysfunction and suffering associated with mental disorder. Chronically starved for resources and outside of public consciousness, the mental health sector persists as a kind of poor relation to other social commitments and without integration into the modern welfare state. It is significant that a comprehensive evaluation of the U.S. social welfare system sponsored by the Ford Foundation did not even identify the mentally ill as a population of concern (Ford Foundation 1989).

Several factors account for this tendency toward exclusion. The expansion of social programs in the United States has followed a pattern of interest-group liberalism in which well-organized and visible clientele groups receive the most benefits (Lowi 1979). Lacking a mass membership and the resources this could provide, lobbying organizations for the mentally ill are a weak political force. The stigma of mental illness also limits the degree to which the general public is inclined to identify with this population. Further, mental health advocates have encouraged the separation of mental health and other social programs by stressing the unique plight of the mentally ill rather than the problems shared in common with other needy groups. The mental health constituency itself has been bitterly divided between diagnostic categories, advocates for children and adults, emphasis on varying priorities such as prevention versus care, and on medical-legal issues such as civil commitment policy. These divisions embody neither good strategy nor sound policy analysis, however. In recent years the emergence of the National Alliance for the Mentally Ill (NAMI) offers better prospects for effective interest group representation, but mental health advocacy continues to be fragmented and weak.

It is difficult to understand mental health policy outside of the larger constellation of health and welfare entitlements whose gaps in coverage affect a variety of socially disadvantaged groups—the high prevalence of uninsurance for health needs and the lack of adequate affordable housing are just two examples. The severely mentally ill are multiply disadvantaged by poverty, disability, lack of housing and employment opportunities, and persistent social stigma. Public mental health care responsive to the needs of a deinstitutionalized system requires coverage of this population within the entitlement structures on which their subsistence and welfare depend. This will require eliminating eligibility restrictions that discriminate against the mentally ill, and repairing the social "safety net" to make it truly comprehensive and reliable. Deinstitutionalization remains an unfulfilled promise. Having initiated policies that keep sick and disabled patients in the community, we require a framework of protections and supports to make the rhetoric of deinstitutionalization less a dream and more a reality.

The Future of Deinstitutionalization

The processes set in motion by deinstitutionalization are unlikely to abate. Regulating bodies and courts have raised the standards for public mental hospitals, and there is less tolerance than ever for indiscriminate custodial care. State facilities also represent a major burden on state budgets, costing almost $5 billion in 1986 (excluding Medicaid). Under fiscal constraints likely to prevail, funding for community programs in many states will depend on further shrinking the public hospital system. New York, the largest system in the nation, reduced the number of resident patients in state hospitals by almost half between 1984 and 1991. The state mental health authority anticipates continuation of this trend over the next several years. Realizing the full advantage of this reduction requires closing some institutions, not simply downsizing the system while keeping existing hospitals intact.

The debate over whether deinstitutionalization is a failure has become a sterile one, not least because the polemics outdistance the data. The question properly requires a multifaceted analysis. Of all patients ever discharged from public hospitals because of deinstitutionalization policies, and of all patients never admitted who would have been hospitalized under previous practices, how many are worse off and how many are better off? How much strain, economic and social, has deinstitutionalization placed upon the community, and how do we weigh the needs and wants of the mentally ill against those of the community as a whole? We have neither the information nor the normative framework to answer these questions definitively. But it simply is not sufficient to concentrate on the most visible deficiencies of deinstitutionalization, such as homelessness, and use them to generalize about the undertaking as a whole.

Finishing the task that has been started will not wait for resolution of such methodological and philosophical quandries. There is little chance of a wholesale return to the public asylum at this point. There is need, however, to provide asylum to a small group of the most severely and chronically mental ill, who are unlikely to ever make a comfortable adaptation to the community or who present persistent danger to society. Accordingly, future mental health policies must develop a comprehensive, balanced care system that links hospital and community services in a complementary fashion. A major obstacle is the traditional value placed on dispersed responsibility within American government. Multiple mental health and other service bureaucracies, operating at different levels of government, limit the coordinating attempts they inspire. One group of solutions, as discussed, pertains to the development of financial and organizational relationships with consistent incentives that discourage fragmentation. Another is to better integrate the mentally ill into programs of health and welfare entitlement in a manner that treats psychiatric disorder comparably to other illnesses. Differential treatment of mental illness in public and private health insurance programs has been a stubborn barrier to access to necessary services. For those most disadvantaged, repairing the "social safety net" to make it more reliable during misfortune should be a basic component of reform.

Arrival of the post-deinstitutionalization era in mental health care has been aptly announced (Shadish, Lorigio, and Lewis 1989). We are now enmeshed in a diverse set of problems focused on caring for chronically mentally ill persons, few of whom have been long-term hospital residents. Some scholars have proposed substituting the label "policies of inclusion" for "deinstitutionalization" to refer to the issues that are attendant on including the severely mentally ill in society (Lewis, Shadish, and Lorigio 1989). The challenge of social integration is daunting, though not insurmountable, and tests the very credibility of the promise of the welfare state. Perhaps the only fundamental mistake of the deinstitutionalization movement was that anyone thought at the outset that this process of reform would be easy.

References

Aiken, L.H., Somers, S.A., and Shore, M.F. 1986. "Private foundations in health affairs: A case study of the development of a national initiative for the chronically mentally ill." *American Psychologist* 41:1290–95.

Babigian, H. 1990. "Capitation financing for the severly mentally ill: Initial research findings from the Monroe Livingston Project." Paper presented at the Third Annual New York State Office of Mental Health Research Conference, Albany, New York.

Babigian, H.M., and Marshall, P. 1989. "Rochester: A comprehensive capitation experiment." In Mechanic, D., and Aiken, L. (eds.), *Paying for Services: Promises and Pitfalls of Capitation*. New Directions for Mental Health Services. San Francisco: Jossey-Bass, 43–54.

Bardach, E. 1977. *The Implementation Game*. Cambridge, MA: M.I.T. Press.

Belknap, I. 1956. *Human Problems of a State Mental Hospital*. New York: McGraw-Hill.

Bleuler, M. 1978. *The Schizophrenic Disorders: Long-Term Patient and Family Studies*, trans. S.M. Clemens. New Haven: Yale University Press.

Bockoven, J.S., 1972. *Moral Treatment in Community Mental Health*. New York: Springer-Verlag.

Breakey, W.R., Fischer, P.J., Kramer, M., Nestadt, G., Romanoski, A.J., Ross, A., Rovall, R., and Stine, O. 1989. "Health and mental health problems of homeless men and women in Baltimore." *Journal of the American Medical Association* 262:1352–57.

Brooks, A.D. 1974. *Law Psychiatry and the Mental Health System.* Boston: Little Brown.

Brown, G.W., Bone, M., Dalison, B., Wing, J.K. 1966. *Schizophrenia and Social Care.* London: Oxford University Press.

Brown, P. 1985. *The Transfer of Care: Psychiatric Deinstitutionalization and its Aftermath.* London: Routledge and Kegan Paul.

Cameron, J.M. 1978. "Ideology and policy termination: Restructuring California's mental health system." *Public Policy* 4:533–70.

Ciompi, L. 1980. "Natural history of schizophrenia in the long term." *British Journal of Psychiatry* 136:413–20.

Connery, R.H. et al. 1968. *The Politics of Mental Health.* New York: Columbia University Press.

Davis, A., Pasamanick, B., and Dinitz, S. 1974. *Schizophrenics in the New Custodial Community: Five Years After the Experiment.* Columbus: Ohio State University.

Dear, M., and Wolch, J. 1987. *Landscapes of Despair: From Deinstitutionalization to Homelessness.* Princeton, NJ: Princeton University Press.

DeJong, G. 1979. "Independent living: From social movement to analytic paradigm." *Archives of Physical Medicine and Rehabilitation* 60:435–46

Dill, A.E.P., and Rochefort, D.A. 1989. "Coordination, continuity, and centralized control: A policy perspective on service strategies for the chronically mentally ill." *Journal of Social Issues* 45:145–59.

Dowell, D.A., and Ciarlo, J.A. 1989. "An evaluative overview of the community mental health centers program." In Rochefort, D.A. (ed.), *Handbook on Mental Health Policy in the United States.* Westport, CT:Greenwood Press, 195–236.

Ennis, B.J. 1972. *Prisoners of Psychiatry: Mental Patients, Psychiatrists, and the Law,* New York: Harcourt Brace Jovanovich.

Foley, H.A. 1975. *Community Mental Health Legislation: The Formative Process.* Lexington, MA: Heath.

Foley, H.A., and Sharfstein, S.S. 1983. *Madness and Government; Who Cares for the Mentally Ill?.* Washington, DC: American Psychiatric Press.

Ford Foundation. 1989. *The Common Good: Social Welfare and the American Future.* New York: Ford Foundation.

Frank, R., and Lave, J. 1989. "A comparison of hospital responses to reimbursement policies for Medicaid psychiatric patients." *RAND Journal of Economics* 20:588–600.

_____. 1985. "The impact of benefit design on length of stay and transfer to residential settings for Medicaid psychiatric patients." *Hospital & Community Psychiatry* 36:749–54.

208   Inescapable Decisions

Goffman, E. 1961. *Asylums: Essays on the Social Situation of Mental Patients and Other Inmates.* Garden City, NY: Doubleday (Anchor).
Goldman, H.H., and Gattozzi, A. 1988. "Murder in the cathedral revisited: President Reagan and the mentally disabled." *Hospital & Community Psychiatry* 39:505-09.
Goldman, H.H., Lehman, A.F., and Morrissey, J.P. 1990. "Design for the national evaluation of the Robert Wood Johnson Foundation program on chronic mental illness." *Hospital & Community Psychiatry* 41:1217-21.
Goldman, H., Morrissey, J.P., and Ridgely, M.S. 1990. "Formal function of mental health authorities at Robert Wood Johnson Foundation program sites: Preliminary observations." *Hospital & Community Psychiatry* 41:1222-30.
Gralnick, A. 1985. "Build a better hospital: Deinstitutionalization has failed." *Hospital & Community Psychiatry* 36:738-41.
Graves, E.J. 1990. "1988 Summary: National Hospital Discharge Survey." *Advance Data from Vital and Health Statistics.* No. 185. Hyattsville, MD: Public Health Service.
Grob, G. 1987a. "Mental health policy in post-World War II America." In Mechanic, D. (ed.), *Improving Mental Health Services: What the Social Sciences Can Tell Us.* New Directions for Mental Health Services. San Francisco:Jossey-Bass, 15-32.
_____. 1987b. "The forging of mental health policy in America: World War II to New Frontier," *Journal of the History of Medicine and Allied Sciences.* 42:410-46.
Gronfein, W. 1985a. "Incentives and intentions in mental health policy: A comparison of the Medicaid and community mental health programs." *Journal of Health and Social Behavior* 26:192-206.
_____. 1985b. "Psychotropic drugs and the origins of deinstitutionalization." *Social Problems* 32:437-53.
Harding, C.M., Brooks, G.W., Ashikaga, T., Strauss, J.S., and Breier, A. 1987a. "The Vermont longitudinal study of persons with severe mental illness: I. Methodology, study sample, and overall status." *American Journal of Psychiatry* 144:718-26.
_____. 1987b. "The Vermont longitudinal study of persons with severe mental illness: II. Long-term outcome of subjects who retrospectively met DSM-III criteria for schizophrenia." *American Journal of Psychiatry* 144:727-35.
Hoult, J. 1987. "Replicating the Mendota Model in Australia." *Mental Health Care & Social Policy* 38:565.
Institute of Medicine. 1988. *Homelessness, Health, and Human Needs.* Washington, DC: National Academy Press.
Kennedy, J.F. 1963. Special message to the Congress on mental illness and mental retardation. *Public Papers of the Presidents of the United States: John F. Kennedy, 1963.* Washington, DC: U.S. Government Printing Office.
Kiesler, C.A., and Sibulkin, A.E. 1987. *Mental Hospitalization: Myths and Facts about a National Crisis.* Newbury Park, CA: Sage Publications.

Klerman, G.L. 1982. "The psychiatric revolution of the past twenty-five years." In Gove, W.R. (ed.), *Deviance and Mental Illness*. Beverly Hills, CA: Sage, 177-98.

Klerman, G.L., and Weissman, M.M. 1989. "Increasing rates of depression." *Journal of the American Medical Association* 261:2229-35.

Kramer, M. 1983. "The continuing challenge: The rising prevalence of mental disorders, associated chronic diseases, and disabling conditions." *American Journal of Social Psychiatry* 3:13-24.

_____. 1977. *Psychiatric Services and the Changing Institutional Scene 1950–1985*. DHEW Pub. No. (ADM) 77-433. Washington, DC: U.S. Government Printing Office.

Lerman, P. 1985. "Deinstitutionalization and welfare policies." *Annals of the American Academy of Politics and Social Science* 479:132-55.

_____. 1982. *Deinstitutionalization and the Welfare State*. New Brunswick, NJ: Rutgers University Press.

Lewis, D.A., Shadish, W.R., Jr., and Lurigio, A.J. 1989. "Policies of inclusion and the mentally ill: Long-term care in a new environment." *Journal of Social Issues* 45:173-85.

Levine, I.S., and Haggard, L.K. 1989. "Homelessness as a public mental health problem." In Rochefort, D.A. (ed.), *Handbook on Mental Health Policy in the United States*. Westport, CT:Greenwood Press, 293-310.

Linn, M.W., and Stein, S. 1989. "Nursing homes as community mental health facilities." In Rochefort, D.A. (ed.), *Handbook on Mental Health Policy in the United States*. Westport, CT:Greenwood Press, 267-92.

Lovell, A.M. 1985. "From confinement to community: The radical transformation of an Italian mental hospital." In Brown, P. (ed.), *Mental Health Care and Social Policy*. Boston: Routledge and Kegan Paul, 375-86.

Lowi, T.J. 1979. *The End of Liberalism*. 2d ed. New York: W.W. Norton.

Lutterman, T., Mazade, N.A., Wurster, C.R., and Glover, R.W. 1987. "State mental health agency revenues and expenditures for mental health services: Trends from 1981 to 1985." In Manderscheid, R.W., and Barrett, S.A. (eds.), *Mental Health, United States, 1987*. National Institute of Mental Health. Washington, DC: U.S. Government Printing Office, 158-86.

Manderscheid, R.W. 1991. Unpublished data. Division of Biometry and Applied Sciences, National Institute of Mental Health, Rockville, Maryland.

Manderscheid, R.W., Witkin, M.J., Rosenstein, J.J., Millazzo-Sayre, L.J., Bethel, H.E., and MacAskill, R.L. 1985. "Specialty mental health services: System and patient characteristics—United States." In Taube, C.A., and Barrett, S.A. (eds.), *Mental Health, United States, 1985*. National Institute of Mental Health. Washington, DC: Goverment Printing Office, 7-69.

Mauch, D. 1989. "Rhode Island: An early effort at managed care." In Mechanic, D., and Aiken, L. (eds.), *Paying for Services: Promises and Pitfalls of Capitation*. New Directions for Mental Health Services, San Francisco:Jossey-Bass, 55-64.

Mechanic, D. 1989. *Mental Health and Social Policy*, 3d ed. Englewood Cliffs, NJ: Prentice-Hall.

_____. 1987. "Correcting misconceptions in mental health policy: Strategies for improved care of the seriously mentally ill." *The Milbank Quarterly* 65:203–30.

Mechanic, D., and Aiken, L. 1989. Capitation in mental health: potentials and cautions. In Mechanic, D., and Aiken L. (eds.), *Paying for Services: Promises and Pitfalls of Capitation*. New Directions for Mental Health Services. San Francisco: Jossey-Bass, 5–18.

Miller, K.S., 1976. *Managing Madness: The Case Against Civil Commitment*. New York: Free Press.

Morrissey, J.P. 1989. "The changing role of the public mental hospital." In Rochefort, D.A. (ed.), *Handbook on Mental Health Policy in the United States*. Westport, CT:Greenwood Press, 93–105.

_____. 1982. "Deinstitutionalizing the mentally ill: Process, outcomes, and new directions." In Gove, W.R. (ed.), *Deviance and Mental Illness*. Beverly Hills, CA: Sage, 147–76.

National Center for Health Statistics. 1988. "1987 Summary: National Hospital Discharge Survey." *Advance Data From Vital and Health Statistics*, No. 159. DHHS Pub. No. (PHS) Public Health Service, Hyattsville, MD, 88–1250.

National Institute of Mental Health. 1989. Unpublished data from Division of Biometry and Applied Sciences.

Newsweek. 1986, January 6. "Abandoned," 14–19.

New York Times. 1989, May 22. Letter to the editor from D.P. Moynihan.

_____. 1987, May 17. "A record prison census."

NIMH. *See* National Institute of Mental Health.

Olfson, M. 1990. "Assertive community treatment: An evaluation of the experimental evidence." *Hospital & Community Psychiatry* 41:634–41.

Osterweis, M., Kleinman, A., and Mechanic, D. (eds.). 1987. *Pain and Disability: Clinical, Behavioral and Public Policy Perspectives*, Washington, DC: National Academy Press.

Pepper, B., and Ryglewicz, H. (eds.). 1982. *The Young Adult Chronic Patient*. New Directions for Mental Health Services No. 14. San Francisco: Jossey-Bass.

Rich, R.F. 1986. "Change and stability in mental health policy: The impact of two transformations." *American Behavioral Science* 30:111–42.

Rochefort, D.A. 1988. "Policymaking cycles in mental health: Critical examination of a conceptual model." *Journal of Health Politics, Policy and Law* 13:129–52.

_____. 1987. "The political context of mental health care." In Mechanic, D. (ed.), *Improving Mental Health Services: What the Social Sciences Can Tell Us*. New Directions for Mental Health Services. San Francisco: Jossey-Bass, 93–105.

_____. 1984. "Origins of the 'Third Psychiatric Revolution': The Community Mental Health Centers Act of 1963." *Journal of Health Politics, Policy and Law* 9:1-30.

Rosenfield, S. 1992. "Factors contributing to the subjective quality of life of the chronic mentally ill." *Journal of Health and Social Behavior* 33:299-315.

Rossi, P.H., and Wright, J.D. 1989. *Down and Out in America: The Origins of Homelessness.* Chicago: University of Chicago Press.

Rothman, D.J. 1980. *Conscience and Convenience: The Asylum and Its Alternatives in Progressive America.* Boston: Little Brown.

Rubin, J. 1990. "Economic aspects of mental health policy and law." In Weisstub, D.N. (ed.), *Law and Mental Health: International Perspectives,* vol. 5, 231-83. New York: Pergamon Press.

Russell, L. 1989. *Medicare's New Hospital Payment System: Is It Working?.* Washington, DC: rookings Institution.

Rutgers Center for Research on the Organization and Financing of Care for the Severely Mentally Ill. 1991. *Evaluation of the Consolidated Inpatient and Outpatient Psychiatric Rate Methodology: Final Report.* New Brunswick, NJ: Institute for Health, Health Care Policy and Aging Research.

Scheerenberger, R.C. 1983. *A History of Mental Retardation.* Baltimore: Brookes Publishing Co.

Schlesinger, M. 1989. "Striking a balance: Capitation, the mentally ill, and public policy." In Mechanic, D., and Aiken, L. (eds.), *Paying for Services: Promises and Pitfalls of Capitation.* New Directions for Mental Health Services. San Francisco: Jossey-Bass, 97-115.

Schwartz, S., and Goldfinger, S. 1981. "The new chronic patient: Clinical characteristics of an emerging subgroup." *Hospital & Community Psychiatry* 32:470-74.

Schwarz, J.E. 1988. *America's Hidden Success,* rev. ed. New York: W.W. Norton.

Scull, A. 1984. *Decarceration: Community Treatment and the Deviant—A Radical View,* 2d ed. New Brunswick: Rutgers University Press.

Segal, S.P., and Kotler, P. 1989. "Community residential care." In Rochefort, D.A. (ed.), *Handbook on Mental Health Policy in the United States.* Westport, CT: Greenwood Press. 237-65.

Shadish, W.R., Jr., Lurigio, A.J., and Lewis, D.A. 1989. "After deinstitutionalization: The present and future of mental health long-term care policy." *Journal of Social Issues* 45:1-16.

Sheets, J., Prevost, J., and Reihmank, J. 1982. "Young adult chronic patients: Three hypothesized subgroups." *Hospital & Community Psychiatry* 33:197-202.

Siegel, C., Alexander, M.J., Linn, S., and Laska, E. 1986. "An alternative to DRGs: A clinically meaningful and cost-reducing approach." *Medical Care* 24:407-17.

Stein, L.I. 1990. "Comments." *Hospital & Community Psychiatry* 41:649-51.

_____. 1989. "Wisconsin's system of mental health financing." In Mechanic, D., and Aiken, L. (eds.), *Paying for Services: Promises and Pitfalls of Capitation.* New Directions for Mental Health Services, San Francisco: Jossey-Bass. 29–41.

Stein, L., and Ganser, L. 1983. "Wisconsin system for funding mental health services." In Talbot, J. (ed.), *New Directions for Mental Health Services: Unified Mental Health Systems.* San Francisco: Jossey Bass.

Stein, L.I., and Test, M.A. (eds.). 1985. *The Training in Community Living Model: A Decade of Experience.* San Francisco: Jossey-Bass.

_____. 1980. "Alternatives to mental hospital treatment I. Conceptual model treatment program and clinical evaluation." *Archives of General Psychiatry* 37:392–97.

Susser, E., Struening, E.L., and Conover, S. 1989. "Psychiatric problems in homeless men." *Archives of General Psychiatry* 46:845–50.

Sykes, G.M. 1978. *Criminology.* New York: Harcourt Brace Jovanovich.

Thompson, J.W., Bass, R.D., and Witkin. 1982. "Fifty years of psychiatric services: 1940–1990." *Hospital & Community Psychiatry* 33:711–17.

Torrey, E.F. 1988. *Nowhere to Go: The Tragic Odyssey of the Homeless Mentally Ill.* New York: arper & Row.

Torrey, E.F., Erdman, K., and Wolfe, S. 1990. *Care of the Seriously Mentally Ill: A Rating of State Programs.* Washington DC: Public Citizen Health Research Group and the National Alliance for the Mentally Ill.

Tyor, P.L., and Bell, L.V. 1984. *Caring for the Retarded in America: A History.* Westport, CT: Greenwood.

U.S. Bureau of the Census. 1987. *Statistical Abstract of the United States: 1988.* 108th ed. Washington, DC: U.S. Government Printing Office.

_____. 1975. *Historical Statistics of the United States, Colonial Times to 1970, Bicentennial Edition, Part 2.* Washington, DC: U.S. Government Printing Office.

Weissert, W. 1985. "Some reasons why it is so difficult to make community-based long-term care cost effective." *Health Services Research* 20:423–33.

Weisbrod, B.A., Test, M.A., and Stein, L.I. 1980. "Alternatives to mental hospital treatment II: economic benefit-cost analysis." *Archives of General Psychiatry* 37:400–2.

Williams, W. 1980. *The Implementation Perspective.* Berkeley: University of California Press.

Wing, J.K., and Brown, G.W. 1970. *Institutionalism and Schizophrenia: A Comparative Study of Three Mental Hospitals, 1960–1968.* Cambridge: Cambridge University Press.

Witkin, M.J., Atay, J.E., Fell, A.S., and Manderscheid, R.W. 1987. "Specialty mental health system characteristics." In Manderscheid, R.W., and Barrett, S.A. (eds.), *Mental Health, United States, 1987.* National Institute of Mental Health. Washington, DC: U.S. Government Printing Office, 14–58.

Wright, J.D. 1989. *Address Unknown: The Homeless in America.* New York: Aldine de Gruyter.

9

Health Care for an Aging Population

The growing numbers of elderly persons in our population are both a challenge and an opportunity for health care institutions. The challenge is to respond appropriately to the burden of chronic disorders that occur with increasing prevalence at older ages, causing physical and social disability and eroding the quality of life. The opportunity is to reshape more completely the pattern of medical care services, initially mobilized largely for the care of short-term acute illness, to one more closely fitted to the burdens of illness as experienced at the threshold of the twenty-first century. Planning of care on a longitudinal basis with attention to quality-of-life issues represents a need not only of the frail elderly but also of the chronically ill throughout the life course.

Patterns of health care organization are shaped by history and sociocultural factors as well as by the imperatives of demography, patterns of disease distribution, medical science, and technology. The health care system is, in its most basic sense, a cultural institution that implicitly incorporates the values, aspirations, and goals of those who organize and provide services as well as those they serve. The development of hospitals in America is a reflection of American society and Western values (Rosenberg 1987), and the extent to which hospitals share so many attributes worldwide reflects in part the diffusion of these values.

Western values put great emphasis on the ability to shape the environment, promoting an active, interventionist approach to disease and, increasingly, to ideas of prevention and health promotion. The public's faith in technology, which shows little sign of diminishing, has facilitated the rapid diffusion of intensive care and new diagnostic and treatment modalities. Such technologies as computerized tomography and nuclear magnetic imaging devices, organ transplantation, coronary angioplasty and open-heart surgery, extracorporeal shock-wave lithotripsy, total hip replacement, and implantation of intraocular lenses are all of recent vintage but make up a sizable component of biomedical effort. These new technologies have special relevance to the elderly population, who are more likely than younger people to have the problems to which these technologies are directed, and thus the elderly account for an increasing component of expenditures.

The elderly are, of course, a large and heterogeneous population with varying types of needs ranging from health promotion and maintenance to long-term care for irreversible dementias and other incapacities. Apart from those limited instances in which science and technology have made possible extraordinary advances extending not only life but also effective function, there are many circumstances in which the challenge for medicine is to facilitate people's abilities to cope with inevitable and often irreversible illness and disability in a fashion that protects the quality of life, and in some instances it does no more than control pain and provide support. The latter challenge may require different treatment contexts, a different mix of personnel, and a different philosophy of care. It clearly requires a longitudinal point of view, attention to the patient's social context, and a broad view of sociomedical needs. While excellent technical care in a narrow medical sense must underlie these efforts, it must be allied with a range of social supports and other services facilitative of coping effectiveness.

The Existing Health Services System

That the elderly depend on and use far more medical and hospital services than other age groups is inevitable with the accumulation of chronic problems and disabilities in older age. The availability of Medicare, which cost $114 billion as of 1991, has substantially increased access to necessary services, but despite the massiveness of the program, it accounts for less than half of the elderly's health care expenditures. The largest gap is in the area of long-term care, where Medicaid, the $119 billion federal-state program for the poorest poor, has become the major funding source, accounting for almost half of national long-term care expenditures. Medicaid coverage, however, is only available once nursing home residents have spent down their assets, stripping many of the disabled elderly of their dignity and commonly leaving their spouses impoverished as well. Recent changes in Medicaid enacted by the Congress provide some financial protections for the institutionalized person's spouse still at home.

The nation spends enormous sums on the medical care of the elderly, but the system of care is highly complex, substantially fragmented, and poorly coordinated. Many elderly people undoubtedly benefit from the sophisticated technologies available to them for diagnosis and treatment, but the system of care is excessively focused on procedures, with too little attention paid to the range of sociomedical issues pertinent to maintaining people in settings they themselves prefer and assisting their coping capacities. Too often, technical medical procedures substitute for carefully listening to patients; assisting them to overcome loneliness, isolation, and depression; and helping to strengthen the social supports they require in the community.

Many of the new initiatives in the health care system are motivated more by the intent to reduce cost than to improve the quality of service. Efforts for case-managed home care were initially organized because of the assumption that avoiding institutional care could more than pay for the additional community services. Most of the demonstrations and evaluations found, however, that it was extraordinarily difficult to target specifically those who were at risk of entering nursing homes and that good community programs attracted new clients with significant need but not those at greatest risk (Weissert 1985). Community care programs were not found to be effective in reducing morbidity and mortality or in cost containment, but they significantly contributed to patient satisfaction and the perceived quality of life among patients and their families (Kemper, Applebaum, and Harrigan 1987). But this, in itself, was not particularly persuasive to policymakers.

Health Maintenance Organizations

Cost constraints also motivated efforts under the Tax Equity and Federal Responsibility Act to enroll more Medicare recipients in HMOs, although there was considerable skepticism about cost savings if significant social selection could not be prevented. A variety of studies had suggested that HMOs were likely to attract more healthy elderly who utilized less care than others (Eggers and Prihoda 1982; Wilensky and Rossiter 1986). It seems plausible that elders who have profound needs

for care are more likely to have established regular and trusting relationships with doctors whom they feel dependent on and whom they are
resistant to leaving. Medicare's experience in enrolling the elderly into
HMOs has been more difficult than anticipated, in part because of the
strong ties patients have to their physicians. Yet, joining such a plan offers
the elderly a broader set of services without the need to purchase
"Medigap" insurance. Although enrollment will be slow, the proportion
of elderly entering such arrangements should increase, particularly as the
increasing numbers of persons who have joined HMOs become eligible
for Medicare.

In theory, HMOs have much to offer elderly patients by managing care
so as to provide a good mix of medical and related sociomedical services.
Because such practice is prepaid, there is no incentive to provide marginal technical services in order to generate income as often happens in
private fee-for-service medicine. Moreover, the elderly are protected
against out-of-pocket payments, which can constitute a significant cost
burden for some of them. For theory to work in actuality, however, the
HMO must be reasonably imaginative in developing appropriate services
pertinent to the needs of older persons and must invest cost savings from
other areas in these services. Without such investments, and a strong
primary-care management structure, HMOs may have little to offer those
elderly who already have excellent accessibility to mainstream care.
There is also, of course, the risk of underservice in plans that are strongly
motivated to reduce cost and be profitable, particularly when physicians'
incomes are reduced when expenditures are high.

HMOs, of course, as an alternative to the existing care system, fail to
address the long-term-care issues that concern many of the elderly and
their advocates. The demonstrations of the social health maintenance
organizations (SHMO) begin to address these issues in a modest way and
define a potential strategy (Hamm, Kickman, and Cutter 1982). Like the
HMO, the SHMO offers a wide array of services within a managed care
system, but it expands the range to include homemaker, home health, and
chore services. Additional services might include provision of meals,
counseling, transportation, and home monitoring, among others. The
range of services may be extraordinarily broad, restricted only by financing limits and organizational capacity to manage and coordinate services
across a range of service sectors. A SHMO may offer these services
directly or may contract with other service organizations for certain

service components, and the models now being tested have varying organizational structures.

Experience in a Medicare demonstration of four such entities suggests that the implementation of this model has been more difficult than anticipated. The idea was to have a single organization provide expanded services to Medicare recipients who would enroll on a voluntary basis and pay an additional monthly premium for the expanded coverage. These SHMOs, covering both unimpaired and functionally impaired elderly were to have a coordinated case-management system to monitor and authorize expanded services for persons who met specified disability criteria. Although the four demonstration organizations studied were able to control utilization of the expanded services and associated costs, they had overall financial difficulties due to acute care costs that were higher than expected, high marketing and administrative costs, and difficulty in recruiting enrollees at the anticipated rates. Three of the four entities did not reach the break-even point until the fourth year, and the fourth is yet to reach this point (Harrington and Newcomer 1990, 1991).

Experience with this demonstration has made some skeptical that the SMHO is an economically viable concept in the competitive medical environments that prevail in areas like those where the concept was tested. However, the problems seem more related to marketing and enrollment than the concept of care itself. The present Medicare environment itself may be out of control, and more stringent cost-containment measures are on the horizon. In this emerging context, it is prudent to continue to investigate models across a wide range of situations that have the capacity to extend the range of care and to allow substitution between sociomedical care and more traditional medical interventions. We have no real alternative other than an enlargement of the nursing home industry.

Case Manager or Gatekeeper

Apart from HMOs, some form of case management is often needed. It is widely recognized that the elderly, given their expected range of chronic illnesses and complaints, could be and often are subjected to very extensive and expensive medical investigations that have limited utility. Moreover, those who are frail but relate to systems of care in an episodic and fragmented way often could benefit substantially from social services, although these are not likely to be mobilized. Thus the importance of the role of a primary physician, who though acknowledged to be desirable in general, is especially essential for those in later decades of life.

Concerns about both the quality of care and the costs of care encourage developing medical case management as a major focus, but, depending upon the emphasis, the manager may be either a sophisticated broker of care or a gatekeeper with incentives to protect the public coffers. Concerns about budgets, deficits, changing demography, and generational equity have encouraged government to seek ways of capitating the Medicare population as efforts to expand cost-sharing among the elderly increasingly confront strong resistance. Moreover, as pressures grow to extend the range of services in Medicare and as long-term-care needs become of greater concern to more of the population and their families, government must be prepared to respond in a framework that offers more control than has typically been available. In the eyes of policymakers, the case manager is more gatekeeper than advocate (Mechanic 1986).

The notion of gatekeeper, one of growing importance to the health care system overall, has special relevance to the elderly, who might be especially disadvantaged in a system that confuses age with morbidity. Very few in the United States would tolerate the degree of rationing based on age that characterizes the allocation of renal dialysis services in England (Aaron and Schwartz 1984), but as pressures on costs grow, reputable spokespersons from public officials to some policy analysts seem to stress the duty of the elderly to forgo available and efficacious technologies (Callahan 1986). Such technologies are sometimes used with poor judgment and with little prudence, but the jump in logic required to ask the elderly to forgo opportunities for benefit simply because they are old is a significant shift in discourse.

Here it is essential to differentiate potential gain from a crude categorization based on age. It is one thing to argue that an individual in a particular state of health and debility has too little to gain to justify a heroic intervention. It is quite another to argue that persons of a particular age, whatever that age may be, by definition meet this criterion. While state of health and debility may be correlated with age, and thus old people may be less likely to be appropriate candidates for specific interventions, the judgment should be made on the basis of health criteria and not on the basis of age.

The Challenges of Long-Term Care

The issue of long-term care exemplifies the intimate relationships between medical care and patterns of culture and social relationships. The demand for such care depends not only on levels of morbidity and debility but also on household structure, norms about family and community responsibility, and networks of reciprocal obligation (Mechanic 1987). The number of nursing home beds needed and the requirements for formal services of many kinds are related to expectations about housing arrangements, informal care, and community supports. The elderly in Western nations increasingly seek to maintain independent households and avoid dependency on children and other relatives (Crystal 1982). Doing so, unfortunately, exacerbates the risk of dependency on formal care and contributes to the complexity of planning for long-term care.

The issue of formal versus informal care is not a simple one. Although patterns of household structures have substantially changed over several decades, with the elderly commonly maintaining single-person households, family members feel a strong sense of obligation and are willing to assume considerable burden (Doty 1986). In a society in which three or even four generations may still be alive, in which there is extensive participation in the work force, in which extended periods of socialization and education are the norm, and in which many households are disrupted by divorce, assumption of daily responsibility for the elderly may pose major burdens for individuals facing other stressful life conditions and transitions.

Policymakers have been extremely wary of extending long-term-care benefits, in fear of replacing informal services with costly formal ones. It is well known that programs that extend new community services attract additional clients who are not of highest risk for institutional care, but the evidence also suggests that such services are mostly supplemental to informal care and not replacements (Kemper, Applebaum, and Harrigan 1987). There is a high level of need among the frail elderly who are capable of avoiding institutional care but still require much assistance in the community. Public policy that views home-based care as only an alternative to nursing home care is unlikely to be responsive to important medical and psychosocial needs among sick elders. The nursing home is a source of fear and revulsion among many elderly, and most will use all their ingenuity and resources to avoid institutionalization. But because the idea of nursing homes is a barrier to long-term care and serves to ration admission, it is a particularly poor basis for defining the threshold for public responsibility. Available resources set pragmatic limits on how deeply we can respond to need, but the current implication that our responsibility stops beyond those eligible for nursing home admission is arbitrary and difficult to justify.

The Financing of Long-Term Care

Ultimately, the issue always comes down to money and who pays. The population of those of seventy-five years old or older, which now constitutes two-fifths of those over sixty-five, will increase to almost half in the next two decades. Similarly, the proportion of elders who attain age eighty-five has been increasing especially rapidly, and the composition of our elderly population now includes many more persons who have serious problems of illness and disability. All of this, of course, puts increasing pressures on medical care expenditures independent of serious efforts to address needs for long-term care.

There is no clear long-term strategy in sight, as I noted in chapter 1, although a growing consensus is emerging on the need to share responsibility. The elderly as a population are no longer in the disadvantaged position they were in during the 1950s and early 1960s, when Medicare was being shaped, and they constitute a heterogeneous population economically as well as in other ways. Our first responsibility must be to care for those who are poor, but we must also do so within a framework meaningful to our entire population. Without such a framework, it is unlikely that we will significantly respond to the needs of the truly poor.

The program we seek would provide access to those who are most vulnerable and in greatest need but would also protect those in the mainstream and their families from impoverishment resulting from long-term-care needs. It would shape incentives for patients, professionals, and caretakers to seek improved function and rehabilitation within meaningful economic constraints and to reinforce—not weaken— the informal care and supports that currently exist. In examining ways to insure that those without resources receive the care they need, we will have to address the responsibilities of the elderly with greater resources as well.

This is not the context in which to examine the complex benefit structures of Medicare and Medicaid or the gaps that currently exist. While Medicaid is currently the nation's long-term-care program by default, it is unlikely that the structure of this program, by itself, can provide an appropriate response. But expansion of federal programs tied to new initiatives in the private sector and a clearer division of responsibilities between the elderly and their families, government and private insurance can provide a framework for an appropriate long-term program in future years.

Because long-term care typically includes skills and services that are interchangeable with informal care—such as meal preparation, assistance with chores, transportation, and so forth—the potentials for shifting responsibility are large. This results in actuarial problems and encourages cautiousness among insurers. There is now increased experimentation with long-term-care insurance policies (Meiners 1986), but the costs are high and benefits restrictive (Ball and Bethell 1989). It seems reasonable that provision of long-term care will require substantial cost-sharing not only to reduce obligations of third-party payers but also to establish a realistic threshold for seeking formal services that might be met in informal ways. Deductibles and coinsurance must not be so large as to provide serious disincentives to using essential services, but they must be substantial enough so there is no obvious incentive to shift new responsibilities to formal care. An alternative is careful screening for eligibility of services by a sophisticated case manager, or gatekeeper, but such screening is often unreliable and can be expensive if the goal is to differentiate accurately between the elderly with varying levels of need (Weissert 1986). As the judgments become more subtle, and not simply an issue of whether a nursing home admission is merited, there is much need to perfect predictive capabilities. Judgments must be made not only about what people can do on their own but also about the strengths and capabilities of their families and other networks. The criteria, then, are entangled with complex personal and social values and with beliefs about the responsibilities of family members, friends, and neighborhoods. This is, thus, an area of high discretion and vulnerable to arbitrary and unfair judgments.

Possibilities for extending long-term-care insurance are many, including having such insurance as an employment fringe benefit or as an option within a cafeteria fringe-benefit program. If payment for such care begins early enough, the insurance costs can be relatively modest, but it is not yet apparent that younger adults are prepared to pay the necessary insurance premiums. Moreover the portability of such insurance between employers may constitute a difficult technical problem until such insurance becomes more widespread. Alternatives might call for mandatory program participation through Social Security or an approved private insurance policy. To the extent that insurance is optional, we face the typical problems of biased selection of risk and how to protect those who lack the economic resources to protect themselves or who play the odds and lose. Inevitably, government, through Medicaid or some similar program, will have to be the provider of last resort for those unable to provide for themselves. What is less clear is how best to structure the government role and to coordinate government entitlements with private sector insurance and patient copayment. Some people believe that while government should guarantee coverage for the large long-term catastrophic costs, a mix of private insurance with cost-sharing by the patient should assume the front-end risk up to a significant threshold defined either by a large dollar amount or a significant proportion of family income. Others believe that government should assure the availability of front-end services when needed, and asset protection in the case of catastrophic cost should be attained through private insurance. There would be, of course, patient cost-sharing in the use of front-end services. The latter approach is more responsive to the long-term care problem, but we have to develop a coordinated approach to public and private responsibilities.

Common Goals of Medical and Social Interventions

Whatever the policies or issues under discussion, too much debate about the health care of the elderly is artificially polarized by advocates of technical and social care, respectively. The elderly have gained a great deal through advances in technology, and they correctly value the new possibilities that medical research makes possible. The issue is less technology and more the goals of the care encounter and how means are applied to solve health problems.

The appropriate criterion at all ages is to maximize people's capacities to perform their valued roles and responsibilities. Increasingly, we are learning that efforts to prevent disease and declining function are as relevant in the later years as in earlier development and that real gains are possible by maintaining healthful life-styles and by encouraging activity, participation, and skill maintenance and enhancement. A growing body of research suggests that the elderly do better when they can retain valued roles, when they can continue to exercise control over their own lives, and when they can maintain a reasonable level of activity. A healthy regimen might involve some daily physical exercise consistent with the individual's potential, engagement in desired activities, some reasonable contact with others, and some direction over the shape of one's day. Among the reasons the elderly prefer to maintain their own households, and particularly fear nursing homes, is the loss of autonomy and privacy, diminished control over their environment and contacts with others, and loss of self-respect associated with the dependence characteristic of institutional residence. People, of course, differ and have varying needs and wants, but medical institutions tend to err on the side of excessive structure, bureaucratic routine, and client dependence.

Institutional care commonly reflects the management needs of those who administer the facility more than the personal wishes and tastes of those they serve. The organization designed to maintain order with minimal effort reinforces docility and passivity among clients and a restricted range of activities. The more poorly staffed and managed the institution, the more frequently patients are oversedated, spend long hours in front of television sets, or simply sit doing nothing. But the one thing we have learned exceedingly well is that the health and vitality of people is best enhanced by an active, though not overtaxing, regimen that maintains involvement and participation in the affairs of everyday life. The fact that individuals have different needs and capacities, and different tastes and wants as well, makes an individualized management plan essential. Clients must be allowed to do for themselves what they can, although in too many settings staff find it easier and more efficient to do things for them. But an effective staff learns to be comfortable with the disorder of having clients take some responsibility for themselves.

In even the most excellent health care facilities, one encounters an indifference to the most basic amenities of everyday living, such as respect for privacy, appropriate forms of addressing elders, and differing styles and paces of activity. There is little question that maintaining treatment environments that have diversity, that avoid impersonality, and that convey a sense of respect and caring is more difficult than maintaining an orderly and efficient atmosphere. But if our goal is to enhance the lives and functioning of the elderly in their later years, we have no alternative but to create more personalized living environments in both formal and informal care settings.

On the service side, American society has the professional personnel, facilities, and organizational capacity to provide a very decent level of care for older people. With our large and growing corps of health professionals and our strong commitment to volunteerism, we have the essential elements for a creative response to emerging problems. Effective health care—both long-term and short-term—will require major initiatives in social organization and community education along with the medical and social services needed. Through a balance of individual responsibility between the elderly and their families, enhanced voluntary efforts, private and nonprofit initiatives, and an appropriate array of public entitlements, we can provide a meaningful framework that gives the later years meaning and dignity as well as the critical services a decent society requires.

References

Aaron, H.J., and Schwartz, W.B. 1984. *The Painful Prescription: Rationing Hospital Care*. Washington, DC: Brookings Institution.
Ball, R., and Bethell, T. 1989. *Because We're All in This Together*. Washington, DC: Families U.S.A. Foundation.
Callahan, D. 1986. "Adequate health care and an aging society: Are they morally compatible?" *Daedalus* 115:247-67.
Crystal, S. 1982. *America's Old Age Crisis: Public Policy and the Two Worlds of Aging*. New York: Basic Books.
Doty, P. 1986. "Family care of the elderly: The role of public policy." *The Milbank Quarterly* 64:34-75.
Eggers, P., and Prihoda, R. 1982. "Pre-enrollment reimbursement patterns of Medicare beneficiaries enrolled in 'at risk' HMOs." *Health Care Financing Review* 4:55-73.
Hamm, L., Kickman, T., and Cutter, D. 1982. "Research demonstrations and evaluation." In Vogel, R., and Palmer, H. (eds.), *Long-term Care: Perspectives from Research and Demonstrations*. Washington, DC: U.S. Department of Health and Human Services, Health Care Financing Administration, 167-253.
Harrington, C., and Newcomer, R.J. 1991. "Social Health Maintenance Organizations' service use and costs, 1985-89." *Health Care Financing Review* 12:37-52.

_____. 1990. "Social Health Maintenance Organizations." *Generations* 14:49–54.

Kemper, P, Applebaum, R., and Harrigan, M. 1987. "Community care demonstrations: What have we learned?" *Health Care Financing Review* 8:87–100.

Mechanic, D. 1987. "Challenges in long term care policy." *Health Affairs* 6:22–34.

_____. 1986. *From Advocacy to Allocation: The Evolving American Health Care System.* New York: Free Press.

Meiners, M. 1986. "Long-term care insurance: Agenda for further research and development." *Generations* 9:39–42.

Rosenberg, C.E. 1987. *The Care of Strangers: The Rise of America's Hospital System.* New York: Basic Books.

Weissert, W.G. 1986. "Hard choices: Targeting long-term care to the 'at risk' aged." *Journal of Health Politics, Policy and Law* 11:463–81.

Weissert, W. 1985. "Some reasons why it is so difficult to make community based long-term care cost effective." *Health Services Research* 20:423–33.

Wilensky, G.R., and Rossiter, L.F. 1986. "Patient self-selection in HMOs." *Health Affairs* 5:66–80.

PART IV

Conclusion

10

Inescapable Decisions

The Legacy of the 1980s

During the 1980s, attention in health, as in other sectors, was substantially diverted from issues of access and equity. Ostensibly, the compelling reason was the need to contain health care costs, but in the interim the medical care industry continued to grow at an incredible rate with new technologies, profit-making entrepreneurialism, and a strong bias toward action under uncertainty. The notion of economic constraints that set limits on what entitlements were acceptable had different effects on varying stakeholders. It was primarily the health care safety net that suffered, while the health sector consumed more resources than ever before, and at an accelerated rate.

Consistent with the pragmatic politics of the era and financial constraints, policymakers had less patience with humanistic issues or questions of social justice. They did not particularly like to hear that the problems of health, and those affecting disenfranchised groups such as the poor, the homeless, the uninsured, and people with disabilities, were more due to our politics and social arrangements than the personal characteristics of those most affected. It was not that they lacked sympathy with the plight of these groups, although some clearly did, but more that they saw little room to maneuver within the constraints as they were defined. There was, of course, consideration of the needs of the poor and other vulnerable populations, but only within the paradigm of health and health care that prevailed, and only in the context of protecting the strong and prevailing interests that dominated the health care arena.

In the 1980s, many of the optimistic assumptions that characterized post-World War II efforts and the social programs of the 1960s changed

229

radically. There was great skepticism expressed about the potential of social reform and the value of social planning. Opinion makers and the population as a whole expressed less trust and faith in political leaders, experts, and the capacities of government bureaucracies. The view that markets provide the best signals of needs and wishes gained wide currency even when applied to arenas like health that depart markedly from market assumptions (Mechanic 1978). And the types of individualism and promotion of self-interest consistent with these assumptions gained a foothold sufficiently strong to undermine seriously the value of social action that extended beyond immediate interests. There was a debasement of cooperative values and instincts that had numerous ramifications.

In the health arena, the destruction of the social bases of health insurance was perhaps the most serious consequence of these trends. The development of third party health insurance historically was a conservative response to the threat of a governmental system of health insurance (Starr 1982) but nevertheless it sought to define community responsibility for sharing protection across wide sections of the population (Somers and Somers 1961). The concept of "community rating" was social not only in that it involved sharing the risk of the costs of serious illness but it also reflected the value that those more vulnerable should pay no higher premium than others. Insurance, thus, was in a significant sense a community affair. The introduction of the idea of competition encouraged insurers to segment markets, seeking to selectively enroll persons of low risk. It became increasingly difficult for small employers and the most vulnerable and needy persons to acquire insurance, contributing to the large ranks of uninsured persons. The motivation to avoid risk is now so dominant among insurers that persons who need protection the most face the largest barriers in acquiring health insurance. Efforts by states to return to community rating and to prohibit arbitrary exclusions are an encouraging trend.

Inescapable Decisions

The latest statistics for 1992 reinforce awareness that health care costs are out of control, now exceeding 14 percent of GNP, and putting a drag on the nation's economy. Indications are that health care spending will exceed a trillion dollars in 1994, with little evidence that our efforts over the past two decades have done much to slow the upward spiral. Despite the level of spending, the number of problems and unmet needs multiply, creating much anxiety throughout the country. We have reached the point of inescapable decisions.

A new president and administration are now in place, aware of the urgency of addressing the cost problem and of closing some of the incredible gaps in the health safety net. During the election, President Clinton endorsed both managed competition and the idea of a cap on health care costs, but the details of these approaches now have to be appropriately fleshed out and negotiated among the many interests involved. Prior to the election there was considerable skepticism in the health care community that there was sufficient consensus to give health reform a high place on the campaign agenda. But as explained in section one of this book, health reform gained salience because of the evidence of continuing failure to control costs and its impact on the economy, because of the large numbers of persons uninsured and underinsured, and perhaps most important from a political perspective, because of growing insecurity among the middle classes about the viability of their future health coverage (Starr 1992). Such concern, when it begins to affect the average voter, is political dynamite, and it is likely to shape the types of compromises that emerge in the tough political infighting ahead.

Getting agreement on principles is relatively easy compared with working out the details on who will be covered, the scope of the benefit package, forms of remuneration, administration, and regulation; and the dominant modes of financing. Medical care is a large and growing business, a major growth sector in the nation's economy. Some 10 million people work in this arena, an increase of 43 percent over the past four years (Pear 1993). Thus, it touches the interests of large segments of our population who depend on the sector for their livelihoods and economic survival. In many communities, hospitals and health centers have become among the largest employers, providing many of the jobs at entry levels available to disadvantaged minority groups. Major initiatives in health are likely to affect, in important ways, the economic welfare of communities as well as individuals. Much of the public still feels well served by existing medical arrangements and institutions, which makes transforming health care a difficult challenge.

Managed competition occupies a central position in the national debate. There are many versions of managed competition, but its core is a simple set of ideas designed to give consumers incentives to make economical choices among health care plans and to promote competition in efficiency and quality among alternative health care programs. Although the early Enthoven proposal (1977) suggested the use of tax credits that could be applied in purchasing a standard insurance package, current proposals call for employers (or government in the case of the uninsured) to contribute toward a standard benefit that employees could supplement with their own funds should they choose a more expensive option (Enthoven and Kronich 1989). Choice among approved competing plans would be regulated through Health Insurance Purchasing Corporations (or cooperatives), which would have the necessary scale and expertise to regulate the selection process, to deal effectively with providers' tendencies toward risk selection, and to engage in such tasks as quality assurance.

The underlying idea of managed competition is that if individuals must pay for enhanced or less efficient insurance policies with their own after-tax income, they will be more prudent purchasers in selecting among options. Thus, health plans will have to compete aggressively in price and quality to attract enrollees. Enthoven's managed competition proposal also would tax employers who subsidized insurance beyond the standard core policy. Thus, if either employees or employers wish to pursue more expensive insurance plans than the standard benefit they would have to do so with after-tax dollars. Limiting the tax subsidy for purchase of insurance remains a hotly debated issue.

The debate on managed competition, despite its seeming simplicity, is exceedingly uncertain because of the many variations among alternative proposals and the lack of experience in implementing arrangements of this kind across a country as heterogeneous as ours. The public discussion of managed competition has been focused on the most salient problems of concern to the middle classes and the model as discussed pertains to a generic middle-class patient. Simplifications are needed to maintain public dialogue, but in the process the needs of special populations may be slighted. Nowhere in the discussions of managed competition, for example, can one find a careful explication of how such a system might affect persons with severe and persistent chronic illness, physical disabilities, developmental disabilities, or even the frail and disabled elderly. Few have examined in detail how the envisioned reforms will relate to the existing structure of the Medicaid program or to state experimentation more generally (Schlesinger and Mechanic 1993).

Gaining control over medical care costs and extending universal coverage would be, of course, major achievements. But in addressing these major challenges we must avoid the types of exclusions and narrow definitions of benefits that leave some vulnerable subgroups in the population worse off than they are now. This is more than a theoretical possibility; some proposals that advocate overriding state mandates could result in less mental health, alcohol, and drug treatment services than are now available, and integrating Medicaid into a national program could result in a reduction of long-term-care services for persons with chronic disabling illnesses.

Great attention is now focused on health care arrangements. While the changes being proposed will establish a framework of care for years to come, this is only the first stage of an iterative process. Not only do thousands of details have to be worked out within the context of whatever system is negotiated, but we will still have to face the broader issues of the functions of health care in a changing society and the type of health safety net required for those who are most disadvantaged. In thinking this issue through, we need to focus not only on entitlements and scope of benefits but also on the appropriate organizational arrangements and the roles of technology, health care research, and professional education. Even more far-reaching, we will have to explore the implications of the role of socioeconomic factors in health, and whether the vulnerable need not only more access than those more privileged but health approaches that are really quite different.

Thinking about Health Reform

Two crucial questions in designing a health reform proposal concern the populations to be covered and the particular benefits included within the plan. Even if it is assumed that plans will compete on the scope of coverage, a minimally adequate standard must be established. Thus, many interested groups, and each reform proposal, seek to define the specific services to be covered. Since traditional insurance coverage is defined in terms of specific types of benefits and benefit periods, this tends to structure how the issue is considered.

The scope of services that can be covered, however, depends substantially on the mechanisms in place for cost control. If the availability of services or periods of coverage are expanded under traditional insurance concepts, the potential for escalation of costs is high. Thus, efforts to work in the context of a traditional model tend to constrain the definition of medically necessary services and exclude many types of services needed by special subsets of patients. Most proposals under discussion, for example, exclude long-term-care services and provide only limited specialized services for persons with disabling chronic illness, such as the severely mentally ill. Demand is curtailed by limiting eligible services, by required cost-sharing and by various types of limits.

An alternative, and different approach is to define the benefit structure comprehensively but tie such benefits to a managed care system that allocates services within the context of a budget-what I described earlier as implicit rationing. To the extent that triage into expensive services is controlled by a "gatekeeper" and is not simply at the discretion of the patient, it becomes more possible to expand the definition of relevant medical services. The constraints of a budget help deal with the cost problem, but within budgetary limits clinicians have an opportunity to trade off one type of service for another. Such an approach limits the incentives to provide unneeded services at the margins, but it also raises concerns about the potential of withholding useful and possibly efficacious services. Such constraints, of course, characterize prepaid group practices and, in an expanded version, the Social Health Maintenance Organizations devised to bring a more comprehensive scope of services to the frail and disabled elderly populations.

The ideal, of course, is a system that provides all necessary and efficacious services while minimizing unnecessary and inappropriate care. In recent years growing effort has been devoted to developing practice guidelines, and the Agency for Health Care Policy and Research of the Department of Health and Human Services has made substantial investments in this area. Such guidelines have potential for informing reimbursement decisions within the traditional insurance system and would also be helpful in informing professional decision making within implicitly rationed systems such as HMOs.

Over the long run, we certainly need a great deal more research on cost-effective interventions, but such research at present (and in the foreseeable future) is not sufficiently well developed to be more than helpful at the margins of medical decision making. Most medical interventions have not been rigorously evaluated, and very few have been examined across all the necessary populations and possible contingencies. It will be decades before such guidelines can play a primary role in defining the scope of necessary and efficacious services. Even as research develops in this area, there are many reasons to proceed very carefully.

Good research on outcomes is exceedingly difficult to do and often takes years of effort. But in the long run, such research is our only hope of ascertaining whether expensive and potentially harmful interventions are beneficial and cost-effective. Many invasive and expensive high-technology procedures are used for years before they are rigorously evaluated, and good evaluation can save lives as well as billions of dollars. A major complication in doing such research, however, is that medical interventions are constantly being refined. Research often has difficulty keeping pace with these advances and the rapidity of changing knowledge and technical application. This poses dilemmas in using research as a basis for defining the benefit package.

Practice guidelines must ultimately cover thousands of situations in a highly dynamic practice environment. Given bureaucratic inclinations toward rigidity and inflexibility, we need to carefully devise a system that is flexible and adaptive to changing conditions. To the extent that practice guidelines become embodied in regulation, they may become entrenched and difficult to change, and constituencies that benefit from current practices add further complications to this process. Practice guidelines and outcomes research are useful advances, but they are no panacea.

Challenges to Managed Competition

It is likely that some version of the managed competition approach will be part of health reform. In large part, managed competition remains a theoretical idea, with many details unspecified. A central concern is whether such an approach can modify cost escalation to the degree needed, and skepticism is implicit in the Clinton approach that seeks to combine elements of managed competition with a budgetary cap on the health sector. Few specifics on implementation are available, and the mechanisms to put these diverse items together in a meaningful way are only vaguely specified. My own belief is that managed competition, in the absence of some global budget, offers little possibility of slowing the dynamic forces accelerating costs and particularly the application of new technologies. As noted throughout this volume, the opportunities for new investments are limitless, and there is little hope we can stem the tide without imposing greater external discipline on system growth as a whole. Other Western nations have been successful in doing this, and we tentatively have begun to develop mechanisms within our own system, such as prospective budgeting, fee schedules, and expenditure targets. Our efforts have been halting and without full conviction, but realities shall force us to bite the bullet.

We face an enormous job of public education. People are truly concerned about health care costs, but individuals typically want no stone unturned when they or their loved ones face serious illness and disability. The public has enormous faith in medical science and its possibilities, and has been an avid champion of a biomedical imperative. While, on one level, the public endorses the concern about underdevelopment of primary care, on another they resist having direct access to specialists limited and often seek specialty consultation at the slightest provocation. The public must come to understand the limitations as well as the promises of intervention, and that medical intervention is not always benign. There must be greater appreciation of the risks associated with aggressive interventionism and particularly the injuries caused by the medical process itself.

Closer to the nuts and bolts level, we have no clear plan for structuring managed competition across a population as heterogeneous as the United States, with its range of population density and health care infrastructure. There are models of such structures for certain populations, such as federal employees and state employee groups but they provide limited guidance on how managed competition would apply to the rural poor, persons with special problems such as the disabled, and other significant subgroups. We have no agreed-upon scenario for how Health Insurance Purchasing Cooperatives (or Alliances) would be organized and managed, how they would structure choice, and the types of mechanisms for resolving conflict they might devise. Most proposals imply considerable discretion for states or localities as they go forward on these tasks, but enormous ambiguities and uncertainties remain. Whatever the local discretion, and this certainly has to be a great deal, national standards and expectations must clearly guide the process.

The idea of managed competition, and prudent consumer choice, is largely based on the conception of a motivated, educated, and rational decision maker who can weigh alternative options against one another and who can select wisely in relation to future needs and expected benefits. This model fits even the well-educated, middle-class consumer only very crudely and may not fit other consumers at all. There are extraordinary variations in health knowledge and understanding in the population, and these are often compounded by cultural differences, language problems, or problems of literacy, and the oppressiveness of disadvantage and stressful lives. Individuals vary enormously in their sense of personal control and their fatalism, and in their capacities to plan ahead weighing possible contingencies. The challenge of how to provide this diverse population with meaningful and understandable choices, and the types of information and communication approaches necessary, will require a great deal of effort and ingenuity (Sofaer 1992).

In focusing on the model (generic) consumer, the advocates of managed competition leave unanswered how such a program would relate to the Medicare and Medicaid programs and new experimental programs in the various states. The Medicare population has shown little receptivity to HMOs, despite opportunities to enroll, and it will be extremely difficult politically to fold Medicare into a national program that offers less opportunities and flexibility than presently enjoyed. Although leaving Medicare out of a national reform initiative creates administrative complexities, and discontinuities particularly for the disabled population covered by Medicare, few politicians have the inclination to lock horns with the extraordinarily powerful elderly constituency. But Medicare recipients might be integrated on a voluntary basis with incentives to join.

Medicaid doesn't enjoy the same special status and most proposals envision eventual integration of Medicaid into whatever national plan evolves. Medicaid has been growing enormously as a result of new federal mandates on the states, and program cost increased by 29 percent in 1992 alone (Pear 1993), with comparably large projections for continuing increases over the next five years under the prevailing system (Health Care Financing Administration 1992). As the Congress has responded to compelling needs and problems among the disadvantaged by enhancing Medicaid, it has also put increasing fiscal pressures on the states. Medicaid is one of the fastest growing components of state government and it has the effect of constraining responses to other important needs.

The Medicaid Dilemma

Although Medicaid is defined by a national set of standards, it has many faces reflecting its multiple purposes and the variations among states in eligibility, comprehensiveness, and innovation. Beyond mandated services, the federal government gives states thirty-one options and the waiver program under Section 2176 allows further experimentation. Medicaid covers traditional acute care services for eligible persons as well as a wide array of long-term-care services for the disabled and elderly population. It provides the only national long-term care protection we have for poor elderly persons, serves as the core of many state programs for persons with severe and persistent mental illness, and for persons with developmental disabilities. With the devastating consequences of the AIDS epidemic, Medicaid now assumes responsibility for approximately 40 percent of persons with AIDS (Health Care Financing Administration 1992). In many states, Medicaid has been expanded recently to include many medically related social services usually not covered even in the most comprehensive traditional insurance programs. Medicaid has also served as an important vehicle for state experimentation in the delivery of services to especially vulnerable populations.

A major weakness of Medicaid is the large variability among states in eligibility and coverage and in reimbursement of providers, which is sometimes so low as to seriously reduce access to care. Thus, how one fares on Medicaid is in major part an accident of geography, and there are large inequities. For example, average payments per Medicaid recipient among the states varied from $1,354 to $5,423 in fiscal year 1990, with an average of $2,568 (Social Security Administration 1991). The disparities were even larger for the disabled Medicaid population, varying from less than $3,000 a year in Mississippi and Alabama to almost $16,000 in Minnesota (Schlesinger and Mechanic 1993). Integrating Medicaid into a larger national program would reduce inequities among the states, but it would also threaten innovative programs in the more advanced states, which have painstakingly built around Medicaid systems of care that respond meaningfully to the needs of neglected and vulnerable populations with persistent disabling illness. Thus, integrating

Medicaid into any national program requires great thoughtfulness and sensitivity to the diversity of arrangements that exist among the states.

On the programmatic level, several state Medicaid programs have designed benefits that match the expanded needs of persons with chronic disabling illness better than most traditional insurance programs. As I have noted throughout this volume, in addition to reforming the financial basis of insurance we also need to encourage a new paradigm of health care, one more attuned to the longitudinal needs of persons with persistent chronic illness and disabilities. Medicaid innovations in some states have begun to move meaningfully in this direction. In pursuing national reform we need to be extremely careful to preserve these advances as we strive to achieve greater equity.

The 34 million Americans with limitations of varying kinds that interfere with usual major activities (Pope and Tarlov 1991) are a significant population, although a minority one. They are affected by a heterogeneous variety of disorders and, thus, do not have the visibility in the policy-making process achieved by such other groups as the elderly or persons with AIDS, who are more easily identified with a common interest. But persons with chronic disabling conditions are particularly dependent on the medical care system for their successful function and adaptation, and their needs should be central to our thinking as we proceed to develop new health care arrangements.

As I have argued throughout this volume, the needs of persons with chronic illness and disabilities are not unique, and the service configuration they require more truly reflects the future needs of the nation's health system than the traditional acute and episodic orientation. In introducing financing and organizational changes, there is always a risk of solidifying traditional approaches and patterns of care. But such change also provides an opportunity to rethink the patterns of care most appropriate to changing disease trends, the demography of the population, and changing social conditions.

Comprehensive Care

When health experts think of Medicaid, they conceive of two programs, one oriented to acute services and the other to long-term care. Some suggest integrating the acute care component into the newly emerging health reforms, leaving a residual Medicaid long-term care program to serve those with persistent disabling illness. The inference is that acute care and long-term care are separate services that easily can be distinguished. Such a separation is workable in assessing financial responsibility, but at the clinical level the distinction is counterproductive.

Our health care system is organized around episodic care. Most of its activities, however, are focused on patients with chronic illnesses who require a long-term management plan for stabilizing their symptoms and promoting effective function. Long-term care, thus, is not simply a service (such as in a nursing home) but a way of thinking about managing illness over time within the context of the patient's home, work, and community environments. It calls for a comprehensive view of patients' needs, longitudinal planning and responsibility, and continuity of care. It requires considerable effort of health personnel to help patients understand their illnesses and to take a responsible role in their own self-care.

A major role in providing effective care for patients with chronic illness is to determine the appropriate levels and mix of services across a relatively comprehensive range of possibilities. Ideally, the practitioner should consider trade-offs between expensive medical modalities and other types of medically related services that help the patient get over difficult episodes and that protect their continued functioning. Some state Medicaid programs have incorporated such services as case management, homemaker services, home health aid services, residential services, respite care, and the like.

A core issue is whether we view health care as a narrowly defined set of remunerated services or as a comprehensive range of services available to a case manager who attempts to devise an appropriate and cost-effective mix. If the former, then the system will be biased toward remunerative services, and the current inpatient bias will remain strong. In contrast, if a broad and flexible set of benefits are financed under a capitated system, there are significant incentives for substituting expanded community services for more traditional clinic and inpatient services. Thus, I favor a broadly defined range of benefits akin to the scope found in the most innovative Medicaid plans but only in case-managed capitated systems. Providing such a broad range of benefits on an open-ended basis would court financial disaster.

There are, of course, many issues that must be addressed in implementation. We need mechanisms to develop the case-management infrastructure that will facilitate thoughtful chronic disease management. One possibility is to expand the long-term care capacities of existing HMOs as in the SHMO demonstrations. An alternative is to develop specialized chronic care providers who contract with primary HMOs to provide additional services to selected patients. It may be feasible to develop specialized HMOs for particular populations who require sustained specialized services, such as persons with persistent mental illness, where the general HMO becomes a secondary provider for basic medical care (Mechanic and Aiken 1989).

The Larger Context of Health Care Reform

The individualistic ethic, pervasive in so much of American life, affects how broadly health issues are seen. Much of the current focus in public health is on seeking solutions to major health risks by urging individual responsibility and personal health action, as compared with social and environmental remedies that address key health risks at their source. Unrealistic expectations about the potential of individual health decisions to determine future health are pervasive. There is little doubt of the value of encouraging people to refrain from smoking, substance abuse, poor nutritional habits, and inactivity. But there is a naive conviction about the ease with which such changes can be accomplished. In contrast, there is little appreciation of the extent to which life imperatives and social opportunities and constraints either enhance or inhibit harmful personal behaviors (Mechanic 1990a). Relative to personal behavior change, such alternatives as improving the safety of living conditions, developing preventive technologies, and devising tax and regulatory incentives that encourage positive health action receive too little emphasis.

This is not to suggest that there has been no progress at the social level. In many areas affected groups have organized to change expert conceptions, and those of the public, of their particular dilemmas. Perhaps most dramatic, symbolized by the passage of the Americans with Disabilities Act of 1989, has been the success of persons with disabilities in conveying politically that the loss of function connected with their impairments is as much a product of social barriers and restricted opportunities as it is due to inherent limitations. Families of the mentally ill, angry at facile psychodynamic theorizing by professionals blaming them for contributing to the disabilities of their family members, have organized nationally and are significantly altering the ways professionals relate to families. Mothers Against Drunk Driving (MADD) has put notable pressure on local law enforcement agencies to enforce existing statutes and has helped redefine public conceptions of the priority of this problem. Various groups have successfully lobbied to change the regulations affecting smoking in public places and have contributed to a significant change in social norms. Major social movements, such as those for women's liberation and gay rights, have significantly contributed to reconceptualizing the nature of the barriers these groups face—primarily defined as personal and health problems—to issues of discrimination and blocked opportunities.

While it may seem tangential to decisions about reform, it is essential to examine deeply the role of health institutions in modern society with its changing demographies, household structures, economic processes, and growing interdependence. How do changing community structures, religious institutions, and transformations of communication and mass media affect the appropriate place of the health care sector and its roles in support and restoration as well as cure? How responsive are health institutions to the new types of health challenges and needs characteristic of modern societies? Given the aging of populations and changing patterns of disease, what are the appropriate emphases on prevention, rehabilitation, maintenance, and caring relative to more acute care orientations? And how might health care institutions more appropriately address the roles of race, class, ethnicity, gender, and age as major determinants of health status and outcomes?

It has been argued that the health care sectors in Western countries redirected their attention to chronic disease as much as a half century ago, as configurations of illness changed with the reduction of common deadly infectious diseases (Fox 1986). While there has been much attention given to cancer, heart disease, and other chronic diseases, the fundamental approach to prevention and care did not radically change, continuing to focus on intensity of service during the acute episode, with relatively little in the way of prevention before the fact or rehabilitation and prevention of secondary disabilities. Risks of traditional illnesses among the young are now small, but the "new morbidity" characterized by social pathologies related to risk-taking, violence, and social disruption take a large toll. Increasingly, we have a bimodal medical care challenge: "new morbidities" predominate among the young, and irreversible chronic disease among the elderly. Since traditional medical care presently offers relatively little in dealing with social morbidities, health care systems have become predominantly highly technologically oriented elder-care systems. But while elder care is basically a longitudinal care challenge of enhancing function and quality of life, most medical care remains focused on the acute episode rather than on comprehensive longitudinal management.

Many agree that we require new approaches to the population's health, strategies that come to terms with personal, social, and environmental risks and that fit the concept of chronic diseases as long-term developmental processes. Increasingly, we learn that aging and chronic disease are relatively independent processes and that we often mistakenly attribute to aging deterioration associated with specific disease processes. Healthy aging requires intervention early in the processes of disease development and subsequently throughout the life course. Once irreversible illness occurs, the challenge is to maintain function and independence responsive to people's goals and aspirations and not to physician imperatives. Increasingly, we learn that the priorities of patients are often quite different than those physicians believe them to be (Wennberg 1990; Eraker and Politser 1982).

Strong technological imperatives persist in medical care, even when the technical modalities have been demonstrated to be ineffective relative to more conservative care (Mechanic 1990b). Whether this primarily results from the aggressive marketing of the medical care industries and motives of practitioners and institutions to maximize income and profits as some contend (Waitzkin and Britt 1989), or from the decision-making logic that physicians follow in taking care of patients, remains unclear. Certainly, all of these influences are important to some degree. There is need to explore thoroughly how these priorities might best be altered and how to develop incentives consistent with broader social objectives.

Some would think it naive to respond to the resistance to change in medical institutions by advocating more education, given our awareness of the powerful economic and professional forces that keep medical care on its present trajectory. But the fact is that the technical imperative is sustained as much by public opinion and demands as it is by corporate and professional control. Surveys suggest persistent support among the public for technical innovation and application in medical care, and physicians often feel significant pressure from their patients to use these technologies and spare no effort. This is reinforced by the manner in which the mass media report on new technical developments, treating as major news promising indications from new experimental ventures. It is the most educated who follow these developments most closely and demand the newest technologies. Thus, it seems clear that the issue is not only educational level but also the assumptions with which we approach issues of health and disease. Over the long run, changing health care assumptions involves changing culture itself, and improved education is a crucial element. The major impact of education may only be evident in the long course, but changing culture is a long-range endeavor, not susceptible to any quick fix.

Credible opinion leaders are necessary in any major educational effort, and it is inevitable that physicians and other health professionals will retain the confidence of much of the public in matters of health. Changing the culture of medical care will require fundamental modifications in how health professionals approach their responsibilities and the extent to which they feel responsible for the caring as well as the curing aspects of their roles. Sociological studies have repeatedly noted how the structure of the educational process, and the social system of the medical school, impede communication and understanding between students and their educational mentors (Bloom 1971). Students typically enter medical education with humane and caring motives, but increasingly become cynical as they confront the demands of their training programs. In the United States, and elsewhere I suspect, there is deep dissatisfaction with medical education among deans, faculty, and students (Robert Wood Johnson Foundation 1992). The public, also, commonly complains of the lack of a caring attitude. Correcting failures in medical care processes depends more on structural rearrangement of care than on teaching the values of caring more effectively. Developing the appropriate structures, however, depends critically on the attitudes of physicians and other health professionals and their sympathies for the priorities and commitments these structures represent.

In Summary

Many questions are yet to be asked in the ongoing health care debate. The current crisis in health care offers significant opportunities not only to close gaps in insurance and impose greater rationality in how we use our resources but also to rethink what we desire and expect from the health care system. Health reform can either cement into place traditional ways of doing business or begin a process of searching how to better incorporate prevention and rehabilitation and respond more sensitively to those with the most profound needs and vulnerabilities. How we design incentives and reimbursement could either solidify medical and managerial dominance or give a greater voice to the other health professions and consumers.

International experience and historical study tell us that there is no single way of achieving our purposes nor is the outcome of our deliberations inevitable. My own preference, as I stated earlier in this book, is a Canadian-like approach organized around universal coverage, portability of insurance, and the convenience and efficiency of a single payer. But even the Canadian system is simply a financing framework facing the same choices that we must confront as we move ahead. Changing paradigms is neither dramatic nor quick. It requires fundamental shifts in how patients, professionals, opinion leaders, and the general public think. We are at the beginning of a long-range process of considering the shape of the health care system of the twenty-first century and the notions of equity and fairness that will prevail.

References

Bloom, S. 1971. "The medical school as a social system: A case study of faculty-student relations." *Milburn Memorial Fund Quarterly* 49, entire issue (part II).

Enthoven, A. 1977, September 22. Memorandum for Secretary Califano on National Health Insurance. Stanford University School of Business.

Enthoven, A., and Kronick, R. 1989. "A consumer-choice health plan for the 1990s." *New England Journal of Medicine* 320:29-37.

Eraker, S.A., and Politser, P. 1982. "How decisions are reached: Physician and patient." *Annals of Internal Medicine* 97, 262-68.

Fox, D. 1986. *Health Policies, Health Politics: The British and Amerian Experience, 1911-1965.* Princeton: Princeton University Press.

Health Care Financing Administration. 1992, July. *A Statistical Report on Medicaid.* Mimeo.

Mechanic, D. 1990a. "Promoting health." *Society* 27:16-22.

_____. 1990b. *Painful Choices.* New Brunswick, NJ: Transaction Publishers.

_____. 1978. "The medical marketplace and its delivery failures." In Weisbrod, B. (ed.), in collaboration with Handler, J.F., and Komesar, N.K., *Public*

Interest Law: An Economic and Institutional Analysis. Berkeley: University of California Press.

Mechanic, D., and Aiken, L.H. (eds.). 1989. *Paying for Services: Promises and Pitfalls of Capitation.* New Directions for Mental Health Services. San Francisco: Jossey-Bass.

Pear, R. 1993, January 5. "Health-care costs up sharply again, posing new threat." *New York Times,* p. A1.

Pope, A., and Tarlov, A. (eds.). 1991. *Disability in America.* Washington, DC: National Academy Press.

Robert Wood Johnson Foundation Commission on Medical Education, 1992. *Medical Education in Transition.* Princeton, NJ: Robert Wood Johnson Foundation.

Schlesinger, M., and Mechanic, D. 1993. "Challenges for managed competition from chronic illness." *Health Affairs.* Supplement:123–137.

Social Security Administration. 1991. *Social Security Bulletin, Annual Statistical Supplement.* Washington, DC: Department of Health and Human Services, table 7.H.1.

Sofaer, S. 1992, December 17. "Consumer protection under health care reform and cost control: Potential threats; potential penalties." Testimony to the Committee on Labor and Human Resources, United States Senate, 231–51.

Somers, H.M., and Somers, A.R. 1961. *Doctors, Patients, and Health Insurance.* Washington, DC: Brookings Institution.

Starr, P. 1992. *The Logic of Health-Care Reform.* Knoxville, TN: Whittle Direct Books.

_____. 1982. *The Social Transformation of American Medicine.* New York: Basic Books.

Waitzkin, H., and Britt, T. 1989. "Changing the structure of medical discourse: Implications of cross-national comparisons." *Journal of Health and Social Behavior* 30:436–49.

Wennberg, J. 1990. "Outcomes research, cost containment, and the fear of health care rationing." *New England Journal of Medicine* 323:1201–4.

Appendixes

Appendix A

Medical Sociology: Some Tensions between Theory, Method, and Substance

The emergence of sophisticated quantitative methods is perhaps the most important advance in the social and behavioral sciences in the past several decades, but progress has been more focused on analytic approaches than on the types and quality of data on which we depend. It is now not uncommon to find talented researchers in mid-career who have never had the experience of designing their own study or gathering new data. Instead, they may depend on the wealth of secondary information available from large-scale surveys. Such secondary analysis is often efficient, and typically provides analysts with larger and higher-quality samples than they are likely to acquire on their own, but by separating the process of collecting data from its analysis the investigator is often distanced from the phenomena under study.

As quantitative multivariate methodologies have come to dominate research work in medical sociology, investigators have split into two cultures, separating quantitative and qualitative studies. These cultures share little communication, publish in different journals, and, for the most part, ignore and sometimes belittle each other's research contributions. In a previous paper I examined discrepancies between quantitative and qualitative studies of medical utilization in order to assess why large-scale multivariate surveys suggested such trivial illness behavior differences while more intensive studies found illness definitions and alternative meanings to be highly important (Mechanic 1979a). I attributed these gaps more to problems in conceptualization and measurement than to an intrinsic incompatibility between methods, and I argued for careful design and measurement tied to the theoretical models being examined. I suggested that combining the strengths of both types of

249

methods provided the most constructive long-term strategy for doing medical sociology. In this Appendix I expand the discussion of dilemmas surrounding the use of alternative methods.

Goffman's Asylums: An Illustration

In 1961 Erving Goffman published *Asylums*, a series of essays based on his fieldwork at St. Elizabeths Hospital, a federal institution housing some seven thousand patients in Washington, DC (Goffman 1961). The book, issued as a paperback by Anchor Books, was enormously popular and was widely cited. Goffman's essays, in association with many other influences, played a significant role in the delegitimation of the mental hospital and contributed to a growing movement in the 1960s to deinstitutionalize the mentally ill. Along with Kesey's *One Flew over the Cuckoo's Nest* and the writings of Thomas Szasz, Goffman helped portray mental hospitalization as a humiliating experience that stripped individuals of their identity and self-esteem and induced a variety of deviant adaptations that were reactions to institutional life. This critique of the mental hospital, embodied within a creative and intriguing theory of total institutions and self-identity, captured the imagination of much of the informed public well beyond the sociological community.

It is unlikely that events would have been much different had Goffman not written *Asylums*. Deinstitutionalization was a product of many influences that extended far beyond the critique of mental hospital care (Mechanic 1989). A democratic and preventive care ideology evolved out of experience during the Second World War, advocating early treatment in the community and a rejection of coercive interventions. The introduction of neuroleptic drugs in the middle 1950s not only allowed control of the most bizarre and disconcerting symptoms of psychosis but also gave administrators and families confidence that patients could be managed in the community. Mental health litigation and the attack on involuntary civil commitment made it more difficult to use coercion to keep patients in hospitals. The expansion of the welfare state in the middle 1960s—particularly Medicaid, disability insurance, and housing assistance—made it possible to relocate patients from mental hospitals to the community and to develop alternatives to mental hospitalization for new patients. Moreover these new federal programs provided states with strong incentives to relocate patients to community settings so as to shift costs from the state to federal programs. Within this confluence of forces, the delegitimation of hospital care was probably important but not crucial. Thus Goffman's work had only a subsidiary role in the massive changes in mental health policy, but it was as influential as any theoretical statement or study can hope to be. It influenced the way many people perceived mental hospitals and contributed to the overall climate of opinion essential to social change.

Quite apart from Goffman's influence is the issue of the accuracy of his critique. Numerous studies using patient surveys, have been done relevant to Goffman's depiction of the experience of the mental patient. None of these studies has the theoretical brilliance of Goffman's work or the quality of his insight, but they consistently fail to replicate his view of the patient's experience (Linn 1968a, 1968b; Weinstein 1979, 1983). Most patients did not report feeling betrayed; many reported being helped by hospitalization, and viewed the hospital as a refuge from impossible problems and stresses. Moreover, some patients from disadvantaged backgrounds viewed the hospital experience as less coercive and less depriving than their usual life situation. The studies do provide evidence of stigma associated with mental illness but negate the profoundly negative conception of the experience depicted by Goffman.

The issue, however, is not simply one of deciding whether the studies based on patient interviews and questionnaires support or disconfirm Goffman. It becomes necessary to inquire more deeply whether this type of evidence invalidates the theoretical "ideal type" of mental hospitalization that Goffman developed. It seems clear that there are strong arguments on both sides; Goffman and his critics may be plumbing different levels and types of meaning with their respective methods.

As an observer, Goffman brought to the hospital his own personal biography and assumptions, which shaped how he saw events. To a middle-class, independent-minded professor, who strongly valued personal autonomy and the right to be eccentric, the regimentation of the mental hospital must have looked repressive indeed. Later in Goffman's life, after he had to live through an episode of mental illness involving another person close to him, he is said to have remarked that had he been writing *Asylums* at that point, it would have been a very different book.

The qualitative observer is, in a sense, a research instrument, and how he or she is calibrated is an issue of some importance. I began my hospital fieldwork in the middle 1950s shortly after the introduction of neuroleptic drugs. Although I had visited some mental institutions during my college years, my first intensive exposure was at Agnew State Hospital in California in 1956. In 1961, when I initiated the medical sociology and mental health training program at the University of Wisconsin, I required that trainees spend a semester as visiting interns at Mendota State Hospital, a state mental hospital. It was clear to me that mental illness and the professional care of the mentally ill were a longitudinal experience, and that short cross-sectional views could be highly misleading. If students wanted to do serious work in the area, they had to become familiar with the longitudinal experiences of patients and the types of challenges they posed to staff. When students first went to the state hospital, they often came back convinced that many of the patients were not mentally ill and were inappropriately hospitalized. As they spent extended periods in the hospital they usually learned that "mental conditions" were more complex than they initially believed, and that patients who appeared normal at one point in time could be highly disturbed on other occasions.

Beginning with my fieldwork in hospitals in 1956, I was impressed by the dramatic improvement in conditions in these institutions during the next two decades. As patient populations decreased, as staff ratios improved, and as hospitals substantially increased their treatment and rehabilitation programs, the mental hospital became an entirely different type of institution than it was in the 1950s. Yet as each subsequent cohort of graduate students took part in their internship experience at the state hospital, they returned with anecdotes documenting what a repressive place it was, consistent with their theoretical dispositions favorable to labeling theory. Not having any basis for comparison with mental hospital care in prior periods, they were calibrated as observers somewhat differently from me.

This point suggests the difficult question of how qualitative researchers, using themselves as a research instrument, properly calibrate themselves. What the researcher selects as important from an almost infinite number of possible observations, and how each observation is weighed relative to others in a larger organizing frame of reference, determine to a major extent the construction that emerges. The way such conceptualization and organization of observations take place depends substantially on the social biography of the observer.

This would seem to suggest the superiority of standardized questions or observations elicited from a representative target group, but this approach also has serious limitations. Any experienced researcher knows that how one frames a question and selects response categories substantially affects the answers received. Respondents to such questions may have difficulties in recall, may wish to withhold important information, or may wish to present themselves in a particular way contrary to the facts (Marquis and Cannell 1971; Mechanic and Newton 1965). The responses may also depend on the order and format of questioning, the timing of questioning relative to the event being asked about, and the respondent's involvement in the interviewing process. In many surveys, respondents are only superficially involved, are poorly instructed, or not particularly motivated to recall accurately, and may respond at a level that fails to reveal deeper feelings and concerns. Thus, although the survey method may seem more objective on the surface, it confronts problems comparable in importance to those characteristic of the qualitative approach.

None of this is to suggest that good practitioners of both types of methods are not aware of these problems and do not make serious efforts to take them into account in the way they design studies or collect relevant data. We have many relevant methodological studies, and some solutions to such problems as acquiescence, social desirability effects, format biases, recall difficulties, and many more, but the complexity of these issues means that in the average study most of these cautions are acknowledged but ignored.

In Goffman's essay on the moral career of the mental patient he depicts in a sequential form how the understandings of the prepatient are likely to be betrayed through the process of referral and admission. Goffman suggests that the prepatient passes through a "'betrayal funnel" with at least a portion of the rights, liberties, and satisfactions of the civilian and ends up on a psychiatric ward stripped of almost everything (Goffman 1961:140). In efforts to examine Goffman's assertions concretely, Linn (1968b) asked 185 patients, most within forty-eight hours of their hospital admission, questions specifically addressed to Goffman's observations. For example, when Linn asked patients "if they felt they have been betrayed by any of their friends or family in coming to the hospital," 75 percent of the patients denied feeling betrayed.

Linn views the discrepancy between his findings and those of Goffman as resulting primarily from sampling problems and the tendency of observers to give undue influence to more interesting, articulate, and novel responses. He acknowledges that his own results based on direct questions to patients could have been shaped by defensive adaptations to their circumstances, but rejects this idea as an adequate explanation of the highly divergent findings. Then again, it is not clear how one establishes how influential defensive adaptive needs may be in shaping responses. In any case, the issues cut more deeply than this comparison suggests.

In an intriguing review of the effects of diet on psychological state, Wadden, Stunkard, and Smoller (1986) found that none of the existing sixteen studies that measured psychological state in a pre-post test design using standardized measures showed any adverse emotional effects of treatment, while all eight studies that used clinical measures reported adverse reactions. Unlike the standardized approach, the clinical observations, although unsystematic, were made at varying points in the treatment process and took account of a wide range of emotional distress. The standardized measures, in contrast, were more specific, were administered less frequently, and covered a narrower range of reactions. The authors conclude that the "method of assessment shapes reports of mood changes during weight reduction and provides perhaps the single best explanation of the contradictory findings concerning dieting and depression" (p. 432). After examining these very different patterns of results, and the relation of results to methods, they suggest that these alternative modes of assessment actually address different questions. Studies depending on a pre-post test design assess the effects of weight loss on mood, while continuous measurement speaks to the impact of dieting on mood.

Wadden and associates conclude, "In the final analysis, we may not have access to . . . 'truth.' The nature of the emotional reactions reported appears to be inextricably tied to the method by which these reactions are assessed" (p. 438). This conclusion is too pessimistic, given the authors' observation that the two sets of studies address different questions. Much of the discrepancy could probably be resolved by more comprehensive specification of the mood states to be covered by standard measures and more frequent measurement during the course of treatment. Such measurement might be impractical for many clinical situations and might pose analysis problems, but it is not an impossible alternative in many situations.

Some of the method differences presumably could be reduced by comparable sampling, consistent frequency of measurement, and clearer specification of definitions and criteria. A more difficult set of issues, however, concerns the validity of what respondents report when questioned directly versus measurement through unobtrusive measures. Direct measures may lack validity not only because of a conscious desire to deceive but also because people's needs may distort their awareness. It is widely recognized that individuals are frequently unaware of factors affecting their decisions and actions, even when questioned immediately after an important event. In experimental studies of behavior, subjects will contest having been influenced by factors successfully manipulated by the experimenter, even when they are informed of the manipulations (Nisbett and Wilson 1970). Goffman's observations appear credible despite disconfirmation by surveys, because readers of his analysis find his depiction meaningful and convincing when they view themselves as the hypothetical patient in the context he describes. Thus Goffman conveys a certain kind of "truth" that cannot be dismissed easily. This type of contextual credibility is often persuasive, having the quality of *verstehen* embodied in the methodology of Max Weber (1949). Moreover, contextual analysis can be adapted in a standard and rigorous way to examine meaning, an issue which will be examined later. First, however, here is a brief review of some of the limitations of surveys.

Some Limitations of Surveys

Much has been written on the design of effective surveys, but the issue here is less concerned with design procedures and more with forms of information acquisition for which the survey is best suited. Survey data are best when the question is clear, and when the respondent knows the answer and is motivated to report it accurately. Some survey researchers view the interview situation as one in which an effective interviewer carefully instructs the respondent as to the information needed and provides feedback and specific cues that facilitate an accurate report (Cannell, Fowler, and Marquis 1968; Cannell, Marquis, and Laurent 1977). In a situation involving repeated interviews, respondents can learn to be careful and accurate reporters. Difficulties arise when respondents do not recall or know the answer to queries; are motivated by fear, stigma, or discomfort to hide or distort important information; lack the incentive to reconstruct experiences in the terms within which questions are posed, or misunderstand the questions. The fact is that demand characteristics of interviews and questionnaires lead many people to answer questions they do not understand. Thus in most such efforts, a significant amount of the information collected is in error. Such error can be minimized through careful specification but many questions on surveys are vague and poorly specified. These problems are compounded by the common use of interviewers with little training and by increasing efforts to contain survey costs.

The quality of interviewing depends very substantially on the credibility and skills of the interviewer. The capacity of the interviewer to gain the respondent's confidence and to guide the patient through the interview affects the data collected. Such confidence may depend not only on demeanor and social characteristics but also on the personality of the interviewer (Cannell. Fowler, and Marguis 1968;Cleary, Mechanic, and Weiss 1981). My colleagues and I found, for example, that respondents reported more psychological symptoms when interviewers were older, more experienced, and when they themselves had low symptom levels (Cleary, Mechanic, and Weiss 1981). We believe that interviewers with such characteristics probably create a more relaxed and more friendly climate that decreases reticence. Such differences are important because we found that some analyses yielded varying results when the data were collected by inexperienced as compared with experienced interviewers.

In surveys we generally assume that respondents will know the answers to the questions we ask. In many instances the questions are too complex to answer without careful scrutiny of records, as in the case of questions about financial assets, details of health insurance policies, household expenditures, and the like. In other instances respondents have only partial knowledge. For example, doctors may detect conditions that they record in the patient's medical record but do not communicate (Feldman 1960). Thus patients may not be able to report completely the diagnosed conditions they have, explaining the discrepancies in part between patients' reports and medical record data.

The issues become more difficult when questions deal less with established facts and more with expected behavior or mental processes. There is an extensive literature on the gap between measured attitudes and intentions and subsequent behavior. Intentions may not result in expected action because statements of intention fail to take account of social pressures, environmental barriers, and motivations that affect implementation. Often people have no clear idea of their own future behavior when unexpected contingencies not considered in the formulation of intention complicate the situation. Usually the question posed is a fairly general one, with no specification of situational contingencies. Although most people will respond to one of the structured response categories, they often know that the correct answer is "it depends." Survey researchers have learned that this is a response alternative that one never offers because respondents will typically choose it.

Some Issues of Measurement

Survey data, when compared to records on factual matters, are often discrepant, sometimes to an unacceptable degree. Part of the discrepancy may be due to errors in the record system itself or to the fact that respondent reports and the records measure somewhat different phenomena. The value of survey data depends on the precision needed. Respondents, for example, can much more reliably report whether they have seen a physician in the past year than specify the actual number of physician visits. If a precise estimate is needed, data based on anything more than a short recall period is likely to contain much error. When the information is less salient to the respondent, shorter recall periods are essential if reliable estimates are to be made. The Health Interview Survey uses a two-week recall period for each respondent, with the sample cumulated over the entire year. In contrast, in measuring a salient event such as a hospitalization or a major surgical procedure, a longer recall period is satisfactory. Even on salient events, a significant amount of misreporting occurs, primarily underreporting. As we ask questions about relatively long periods such as six months or a year, respondents more readily forget or have difficulty visualizing the boundaries of the question. Thus they may identify particular events with the wrong periods. In using shorter recall periods a calendar is helpful, but as one asks questions extending over long time periods, respondents usually need salient life events to locate particular occurrences in time.

Respondents misreport even the simplest items, such as age, and do so in a way that introduces systematic biases. Age, for example, is commonly reported in round numbers (50, 55, 60); middle-aged persons tend to underreport age, and some elderly overreport age (Mechanic 1978a:140-43). As one moves from highly objective items to those requiring a judgment call, reliability decreases substantially. Members of a household show high levels of disagreement on who performs a wide variety of household tasks when questioned in conventional ways, but more thorough interviewing elicits much higher levels of agreement (Brown and Rutter 1966). Poor reliability is not inevitable; if the investigator makes the effort and takes the time to ask questions in detail and in a precise way, reliability can be much improved. Yet few surveys make the necessary investment and accept a high level of error.

In recent years there has been an increase in longitudinal study, which assists in making causal inferences, but most studies depend on retrospective reporting. Such reporting faces two major problems. First, the retrospective reports assessing values on independent variables are obtained concurrently with dependent measures, creating an unknown degree of confounding. Not only is it difficult to assess what caused what, but the answers to the two sets of questions within the interview context may be related in the respondent's mind-set and response pattern. Similarly, proxy data is commonly distorted; respondents often project their own inclinations and needs onto others. Correlations between reports about oneself and about others are almost always higher when the reports are obtained from the same respondent than when they are obtained from independent sources. Second, retrospective reports are suspect because people typically reconstruct their past in light of subsequent events. Not only does time change the meanings and affect associated with events, but people also reconstruct the factual basis of these events. Such distortions in part are a product of recall problems and in part serve psychological needs to maintain an integrated and positive sense of personal identity.

The process of living a life is a dynamic adaptive process in which individuals change in relation to changing circumstances and the particular challenges they face. How they perceive events at any point in time depends on the immediate situation and the relative salience of various elements in their life stories. The point in time at which one cuts into this life story determines the nature of the observations one makes. Qualitative studies demonstrate amply how substantially people's conceptions of their lives are shaped by their needs. One of my favorite examples is a study by Fred Davis (1963), who followed polio victims and their families for several years. Thus he had an opportunity to compare concurrent observations of family life and coping with later retrospective reports. Although Davis describes large changes in family life in coming to terms with polio, families reported little change.

> Throughout this work we have been concerned with the way in which the child and his family came to conceive of themselves as a result of the child's illness, his separation from the home, and his reincorporation into it as a handicapped person. The data appear to suggest a striking anomaly: although it is clear that much was changed in the family, both objectively and subjectively, by these experiences, it is equally clear that the appreciation by family members of what had transpired in no way matched the magnitude of the changes themselves. Regardless of whether, for example, the families normalized or disassociated the social meaning of the child's handicap, the ebb and flow of daily life appeared to remain sufficiently static to leave them with the conviction that nothing had changed, that the child was essentially the same person he had been prior to his illness, and that everyone in the family felt and acted towards the others as he always had.

> It is less important to question the accuracy of such perceptions—that they contradicted certain of the existential realities has been amply documented—than it is to weigh their significance for the organizational stability and psychological continuity of family life . . . the disparity between the changes actually wrought and their reflexive effects on family identity is at the very heart of the question of how a corporate entity such as the family can, in the face of the unexpected, the disruptive, and the transforming, continue to function without breaking drastically from its particular historic identity. (Pp. 175–76)

The Davis commentary goes beyond the issue of retrospective reconstruction. In facing adversity, individuals often have a need to view events in certain comforting ways. Thus, answers to many types of questions may reflect these coping efforts when the subject matter of the investigation overlaps with them (Mechanic 1978b). There are, of course, many types of information not affected by these adaptive processes, but their influence is quite wide.

As the salience of an important event recedes, the affect associated with that event and the memory of it tend to fade. Thus it is comforting for the researcher to assume that reporting errors will simply be underreports that affect precision but not basic trends. This assumption seems consistent, for example, with methodological studies of morbidity and medical utilization. Reports seem to be highly dependent on the length of the recall period. There is some overreporting, but this is never explained adequately and usually is attributed to associating events mistakenly with the period being asked about. We know, however, from our own experience that a salient event can be imprinted effectively in our memory over many years. Very few adults, for example, cannot recall where they were and what they were doing when they first learned that President Kennedy had been assassinated. Highly salient events are usually important ones and some researchers assume that retrospective reports on such events therefore can be elicited accurately. Unfortunately, salience can also result in major distortions.

In an intriguing study of patients who had gastric surgery for obesity, Stunkard and his colleagues (1985) had an opportunity to examine concurrent and retrospective reports on postoperative vomiting. Such vomiting, associated with the surgical intervention of gastric reduction, was believed to be a serious adverse effect, raising concerns about the surgery. The investigators had an opportunity to compare weekly reports from patients on the number of times they vomited each week with a six-month retrospective report on the same measure. Using concurrent weekly measures, the investigators found only infrequent vomiting; even in the first postoperative month, when vomiting was particularly high, the average was only 3.4 times per week. In contrast, six-month retrospective reports yielded rates that were much higher and statistically significant for comparisons of the first week, the first month, and the first two months. The differences were smaller for the later periods. Seventy-three percent of patients reported low rates on both types of measures, but 28 percent reported much higher rates of vomiting retrospectively than concurrently. A two-year follow-up of six of the patients who were high retrospective reporters showed that they continued to make high retrospective reports two years later. As the investigators note, "Once patients had formed an impression of a high rate of vomiting, it did not change over time" (p. 153).

An important lead is the fact that those who were high retrospective reporters lost significantly less weight. The correlation between weight loss and vomiting was -.58, but it was not statistically significant because of the small number of patients. It seems plausible that a phenomenon such as disappointment may have been operative. Persons who went through a difficult surgical procedure but failed to achieve the expected weight loss may then generalize their disappointment by attributing to the surgery retrospectively more adversity than they experienced at the time. In a related finding, Cartwright (1967) noted that British general practitioners gave much higher estimates of trivial patient consultations in their practice than were elicited when they kept one-day records of their patient consultations, and these discrepancies were larger among dissatisfied doctors. In a subsequent study, I showed that these high estimates of trivial and inappropriate patients were more a reflection of the doctors' general dissatisfaction and frustration than of patients' behavior (Mechanic 1970; see also Cartwright and Anderson 1981).

Some Approaches to Closing Gaps between Methods

Research questions should dictate methodology and researchers should be prepared to use a variety of methods that contribute to a deeper understanding, triangulating varying approaches to the same problem. Thus I particularly endorse combining the advantages of the survey (its scope and its sampling opportunities) with the intensity of observation of the smaller qualitative study. They can be used in mutually enhancing ways.

Issues of Time and Meaning: Illness Behavior as an Illustration

Illness behavior can be defined as the ways in which persons respond to bodily indications and the conditions under which they come to view them as abnormal. Thus, this concept involves the manner in which people monitor their bodies, define and interpret their symptoms, take remedial action, and use various sources of help as well as the more formal health care system (Mechanic 1986). This definition should make it clear that the focus of such study is *behavior* that may vary enormously across sociocultural circumstances and in relation to values and situational contingencies. The investigation of illness behavior provides a perspective that helps us understand the inconsistencies between medical rationality and the response of individuals. Such a perspective contributes to a more accurate portrayal of illness processes and possibilities for constructive interventions.

Illness behavior encompasses a range of sociocultural, interactional, and cognitive processes. These processes are dynamic and extend through time. Most studies, however, are cross-sectional, simply sampling a slice from complex chains at a single point. Thus they commonly fail to capture the interactive character of assessments and response, and vastly underestimate the power of illness behavior to shape episodes and the course of illness (Mechanic 1979a).

Perhaps the most common type of investigation is the cross-sectional help-seeking survey, in which efforts are made to predict utilization in terms of single measures of illness behavior, attitudes, predispositions, social stresses, and the like. Typically, recall periods cover six months, a year, or even more. A gross correlation is obtained, properly adjusted for a variety of confounding variables, but in a manner that completely ignores the processual nature of illness perceptions and response. Temporal links between predisposing variables and measured outcomes are almost completely obliterated.

When people become aware of symptoms, they make efforts to understand their implications for their well-being. In the case of relatively minor and self-limited symptoms, this process may be truncated and brief. In situations of uncertainty, however, or in instances of severe and potentially disabling or life-threatening conditions, individuals may go through an extended appraisal process in which they seek to identify the causes of their problem and alternative options for response. These appraisal processes are influenced by the nature of symptoms and how they present, prior socialization and sociocultural learning, personal traits, and situational contingencies.

Such appraisal processes affect not only what people choose to do about their symptoms, but also the significance they attribute to them in terms of their life plans. The enormous variability in response to comparable symptoms among patients has long been a subject of interest. Why do comparable patients vary to such large degree in their complaining behavior, in their propensity to use health care resources, and in the degree of disability they experience? For some patients, the illness or condition becomes central to their daily life and personal identity; for others, the illness and the resulting disability remain peripheral. Patients with serious illness typically can provide an explanation of why they became sick when they did, drawing on many commonly understood cultural themes. How they construe such issues may affect the trajectory of their illness.

Leventhal and his colleagues (1980, 1985) illustrate some of these points nicely in a study of patients with hypertension. Physicians assume, with good empirical support, that patients with hypertension cannot assess when their blood pressure is high or low. Patients, although accepting the general notion, believe that they can. Such patients use environmental cues consistent with cultural explanations to "tell them" when their blood pressure is high or low. Thus they learn that stress is related to increases in blood pressure and relaxation to decreases, and adjust their medication accordingly. When they feel relaxed, they decrease hypertensive therapy, assuming that less medication is necessary. Aware that physicians do not believe that patients can successfully monitor their blood pressure, they withhold information from physicians regarding modifications of medication regimens. Some patients even asked the investigators not to inform their physicians, because of their awareness of the physicians' skepticism regarding these abilities.

The use of "naive" theories by patients in defining and managing illness is extremely common, and reflects the broader processes in social life in which assessments of meaning and intention influence social relations. Such meanings may develop and change as people acquire new information that modifies or disconfirms earlier appraisals. Methods of inquiry—if they are to be suitable—must capture the dynamic nature of these meaning systems and how they are influenced by sociocultural factors and situational contexts. The inconvenience of addressing these issues in the typical survey constitutes the single largest barrier to the further development of this area of inquiry. There are many small patient studies, but they typically lack the diversity and representativeness of large-scale surveys and allow for few controls in assessing causal processes. The use of diaries can be an important link between these alternative approaches.

Diaries

The use of diaries in social research goes back fifty years, but they have been used only occasionally in health research. Experience indicates that they report symptoms and disabilities more completely than other methods and minimize common errors characteristic of retrospective surveys (Verbrugge 1980). If persons maintaining diaries are appropriately instructed and monitored, data quality is high and acceptable levels of cooperation are achieved. For the study of illness behavior and the links among situational factors, stress, symptoms, and health actions, diaries are particularly advantageous because of the alternative opportunities of linking time sequences. In a very thoughtful review, Verbrugge (1980) has examined both the unexplored potential and the limits of diary studies; she has also used diaries to explore a variety of intriguing questions about how individuals manage common symptoms and take health actions (Verbrugge 1985; Verbrugge and Ascione 1987).

Verbrugge reported on 589 respondents in the Health in Detroit Study who kept diaries as part of this investigation. The diary period was six weeks but data were included on all who kept the diary for at least a week. The results are complex and not easily summarized, but they amply illustrate the potentials of linking symptom days, episodes, moods, physical malaise, and health actions. Symptoms, physical malaise, bad moods, and negative events predicted health actions on the subsequent day (Verbrugge 1985). Reinforcing the point made earlier about timing of events, triggers for health action were stronger on the same day than on subsequent days. The importance of such timing considerations in examining the impact of triggers on health actions has also been illustrated by Roghmann and Haggerty (1972) and Gortmaker, Eckenrode, and Gore (1982). Diary studies also show that health responses are specific to symptom configurations. Verbrugge and Ascione (1987), in contrasting respiratory and musculoskeletal symptoms, find that in instances of acute respiratory illness, symptoms mainly dictate health decisions; in the case of the more chronic musculoskeletal complaints, other factors play a larger part in shaping response.

The analytic management of diary data and the identification of appropriate statistical techniques for studying sequences pose important challenges. Yet it seems that diaries may be uniquely suited to capture in a rigorous quantitative form many of the sequential processes that theories of help-seeking suggest (Mechanic 1978a). Most of the work with diaries has been descriptive and inductive, but diaries could also be good tools to examine our theories more closely than has been possible with typical survey data. This method will require careful choice of diary items that present the most important concepts in a parsimonious framework. It is also necessary to be sensitive to possible biases in the use of diaries.

Verbrugge (1980) reviewed conditioning effects on diary data, noting effects of both sensitization and fatigue. She concludeed that "levels of health reporting tend to drop over time in diary studies . . . this suggests that conditioning effects are present. They are not especially large; most indicators drop 5 to 25 percent over a 2 to 3 month period" (p. 90). The drop can be attributed to fatigue, boredom, loss of interest, and the like; in contrast, Verbrugge has little to say about sensitization. Ironically, it was through the use of diaries that I first became aware of the importance of sensitization as a factor affecting perceptions of physical and psychological distress.

In a family health study in 1961, we asked mothers to complete a standardized diary each day for fifteen days following a household interview (Mechanic and Newton 1965). Although we had an excellent response rate in the survey, we did less well in achieving cooperation for completion of the diaries. In retrospect we should have made more effort to insure completion; health diary studies have been able to achieve very respectable response rates (Verbrugge 1980:88–89, table 3). In asking some mothers why they did not complete the diary, we were told that filling out the standard symptom items each day made them feel sick.

In recent years a substantial body of research has accumulated showing that sensitization (as measured by indexes of introspection or private-self-consciousness or self-attention as induced by experimental instructions and manipulations) is associated with increased reporting of physical and psychological symptoms (Hansell, Mechanic, and Brandolo 1986; Mechanic 1979b, 1980, 1983). Such self-awareness may be viewed as a more or less stable personality trait, making individuals sensitive to bodily changes or as situational effects induced by particular social and environmental contexts that draw individuals' attention to internal states. It seems that such states can be relatively enduring aspects of persons but also can be situationally triggered. It is plausible that individuals who are more introspective and more attuned to their bodies and feelings should be more susceptible to environmental inducers, but evidence on this point remains weak.

Introspectiveness affects the magnitude of reporting of physical and psychological symptoms. It may do so in a variety of ways. Persons who attend to their bodies and feelings are more likely to notice untoward states, while those who are distracted from themselves may be less perceptive. Moreover, the processes of attention may amplify the symptom and make it appear more important. Continued appraisal may make the symptom more central or more important in the person's perceptual gestalt, reinforcing awareness. Self-awareness, however, is only one of many possible traits or inclinations that may affect perceptions and reports. It has long been recognized that mood, neuroticism, and other psychological states affect reports, and similarly, such traits as optimism, self-efficacy, and self-esteem may also be important. Thus, in using diaries, investigators aware of sensitization effects could control for differential reporting inclinations, using these measures not only as a check against possible reporting biases but also as an opportunity to enhance our knowledge of these effects.

Contextual Analysis

Most qualitative studies focus attention on the specific context in which behavior takes place. The social survey, in contrast, may make efforts to measure important contextual variables, but typically it separates most behavior measured from the particular historical, social, and cultural contexts in which it is embedded. This explains partially why so much that is measured has low stability and is highly sensitive to changes in the environment. It also explains why multivariate analyses based on survey data commonly explain only a little of the variation in dependent variables of interest. The study of stressful life events is instructive.

The introduction of the Holmes-Rahe scale of life change events made an important contribution to stimulating quantitative studies on stress (Holmes and Rahe 1967). By asking respondents to report whether items on a standard list of events had happened to them, researchers could assign respondents a life-change score, which could then be associated with a range of health and illness measures. The Holmes-Rahe scale, and many of the other life event scales that followed in its wake, separate the occurrence of events such as death, divorce, job loss, promotion, and the like from the contexts in which they occurred. The early scales had many serious deficiencies involving the specification of events and recall periods as well as other issues related to comprehensiveness, degree of desirability or undesirability of events measured, independence of events relative to the respondent's behavior, and the like (see Dohrenwend and Dohrenwend 1974, 1981). Over time, efforts have been made to expand the list and to improve the descriptions of events, to define recall periods more clearly, to measure each event's perceived impact, and to assess independence. Despite these efforts, life-events research continues to be torn from its contexts of meaning and has made only limited advances.

An alternative method, developed in England by Brown and Harris (1978), seeks to capture objectively the meanings of specific events, independent of the respondent's perceptions, by using what they call a contextual rating. Through an extensive semistructured interview, the patient's life story is elicited. Reported events are then evaluated in terms of type and magnitude by trained raters who follow highly developed coding manuals. In establishing this rating, coders make a contextual evaluation of how a typical person in a similar situation, as described by the interview, would construe the situation in terms of its stressfulness and difficulty. Thus this method allows for an objective rating of events independent of respondents' subjective responses but building on the context of the person's life situation. Such coding also allows for relatively precise timing of important events, which facilitates analyses that take into account not only what events occur but also when they occur. Brown and his colleagues have been more successful than many other investigators in developing interesting models of depression and other conditions from these data (Brown and Harris 1978, 1989), although the approach continues to be debated. One major criticism is that raters who use life context to impute meaning to events may take into account social factors that may also be used in the analyses of life events. The lack of independence between the ratings and measures of social factors may lead to spurious findings (Bebbington 1986).

Only one study, as far as I can determine, has attempted to compare the results of Brown's method with the more conventional rating scales. Katschnig (1986) studied two clinical samples: 42 patients in Edinburgh who had attempted suicide and 147 depressed patients in Vienna. Each of these patients received first the Holmes and Rahe self-rating list and then Brown's Life Event and Difficulty Scale (LEDS) after the depressive episode had ended, so as to minimize the possibility that depressed mood would influence recall. In the latter case, life events were classified by Brown's method. Using grouped data, Katschnig found that the two methods yielded very similar results, linking life events to outcome measures. When global stress scores among individual patients were compared, comparability was diminished but similarities persisted. Yet, when one examines the specific individual events elicited by the two methods for the same respondents, there is almost no overlap at all. Katschnig concludes that "life event methods do in fact differ from one another in many respects and that 'similar' results obtained with different methods are deceptive. It was shown that it is not possible to dispense with the detailed collection of information on life events and their context. It would therefore be wise to refrain from continuing to use self-rating checklists with predetermined life stress values" (Katschnig 1986:103–4).

This issue, which is rediscovered again and again in varying ways, was addressed by Paul Lazarsfeld (1959), who maintained that underlying classificatory efforts were latent properties on which people differed. Measurement, as a method to capture the underlying imagery or latent properties, involves a large possible universe of indicators of which the investigator will use only a subset. As Lazarsfeld noted, "All indicators are related to an intended underlying classification only with a probability" (p. 62). He further suggested, "If we have a reasonable collection of indicator items, then for most purposes it does not matter much which subset we use to form our index. This is true so long as our aim is to find statistical relations among a number of variables, not the correct classification of each person" (p. 62). Lazarsfeld noted that even when the indicators were not highly correlated, they usually produced the same result when related to an outside variable. Lazarsfeld then stated what he called the rule of the "interchangeability of indices":

> To translate a rather broad but non-specific concept into an empirical research instrument, there will always be a large number of indicators eligible for a classificatory index. A relatively small number of such items is practicably more manageable. If we choose two sets of reasonable items to form two alternative indices, we will usually find that (1) the two indices are related, but they do not classify all the people in a study in precisely the same way; and (2) the two indices lead to similar empirical results if they are separately cross-tabulated with a third, "outside" variable. (P. 64)

Lazarsfeld's rule typically holds in studies of stressful life events; however such events are measured, scored, and weighted, they commonly yield the same general result linking adverse life events to psychological and physical morbidity. All of these measures appear to capture, in one way or another, the degree of disorganization and disruption in the person's life circumstances. Such measurement, however, does not take us very far because the aggregate association is not particularly interesting. We can make appropriate advances only by knowing what types of events under what circumstances lead to what specific outcomes. It is at this specific level that the various rating scales, as now constituted, seem wanting relative to a method that defines events carefully (not leaving definition to the discretion of each respondent), that carefully distinguishes events from the psychological states with which they are commonly correlated, and that places these events more precisely in time and context. Brown's method is more time-intensive, expensive, and is not free of possible contamination, but it approximates much more closely the degree of conceptual clarity and specificity essential to achieving deeper understanding.

A Social Theory of Data

In an important and provocative book, Lieberson (1985) examines the ways in which sociologists typically misuse multivariate techniques and the need to tie data collection and analysis more closely with theory development. He maintains that more effort should be given to understanding why phenomena exist, in contrast to explaining variations in their occurrence. Moreover, he argues, the ritualistic explanation of the maximal amount of variance, which confuses major causes with non-generalizable variations due to situation, time, or sampling, misfocuses our efforts. Many of Lieberson's criticisms can be thought of in terms of model misspecifications (Arminger and Bohrnstedt 1987), but he identifies vividly how technical developments sometimes have diverted researchers from fundamental inquiry.

Lieberson argues for a theory of data, one that bears on the specific problems addressed. As he notes:

> If comparisons are made, we cannot assume that it is mere chance that some comparative possibilities exist and others do not. . . . Likewise, if measurements are made, we cannot assume that it is by chance that certain times and places allow for such measurements and others do not. If we want to study the influence of a new force, we cannot assume that it is by chance that it operates now and not at some other time. . . . Now, this too means that the social conditions of interest are also determining the data available as much as anything else does. (1985:229–30)

Many of the problems in medical sociological research, as illustrated by some of the examples I have presented here, result from a lack of theory about our data and their meaning. Sociologists, including Lieberson, generally emphasize the analysis phases, giving much less attention to how data are generated and what answers to questions mean within the cognitive framework of the respondent and the shared conceptual system of a social group. We now know that logically comparable questions, framed differently, yield varying preferences (Tversky and Kahneman 1974), and there is growing interest in the connections between survey work and cognitive theory (Fienberg, Loftus, and Tanor

1985). Enhanced understanding in these areas is likely to improve our efforts.

Much of the substance of sociology is assortative processes and these should be a major focus of our attention (Mechanic 1975). Many of our methodological efforts are directed at eliminating selective effects through experimentation or controlling them through statistical manipulations. It is important to do so, but not at the cost of forgetting that much of human behavior and many social processes are governed by the conditions that produce selection. In discussing the technology of adjusting selection bias, Singer and Marini (1987) argue that "a more productive activity would first involve a shift of philosophy in which selection processes as such are viewed as primary foci of investigations" (p. 388).

In our efforts to understand our world around us we recognize many technical barriers, but we use the best methods we can. We have, in fact, made enormous progress in almost every aspect of data collection and analysis, but it does us well to reexamine our assumptions periodically and to inquire more deeply about the meaning of the information that serves as a source of our interpretations of reality. By inquiring more carefully about what the data mean, we can also bridge gaps between the research cultures of those committed to varying types of methods.

References

Arminger, G., and Bohrnstedt, G.W. 1987. "Making it count even more: A review and critique of Stanley Lieberson's *Making it Count: The Improvement of Social Theory and Research*." In Clogg, C.C. (ed.) *Sociological Methodology*, vol. 17, 366–72. San Francisco: Jossey-Bass.
Bebbington, P. 1986. "Establishing causal links—recent controversies." In Katschnig, H. (ed.), *Life Events and Psychiatric Disorders: Controversial Issues*. Cambridge: Cambridge University Press, 188–200.
Brown, G., and Harris, T. (eds). 1989. *Life Events and Illness*. New York: Guilford Press.
———. 1978. *Social Origins of Depression: A Study of Psychiatric Disorder in Women*. New York: Free Press.
Brown, G.W., and Rutter, M. 1966. "The measurement of family activities and relationships: A methodological study." *Human Relations* 19:241–63.
Cannell, C.F., Fowler, F.J. Jr., and Marquis, K.H. 1968. "The influence of interviewer and respondent psychological and behavioral variables." *Vital and Health Statistics*, ser. 2, no. 26. Rockville, MD: National Center for Health Statistics.

Cannell, C.F., Marquis, K.H., and Laurent, A. 1977. "A summary of studies of interviewing methodology." *Vital and Health Statistics*, ser. 2, no. 69. Rockville, MD: National Center for Health Statistics.

Cartwright, A. 1967. *Patients and Their Doctors: A Study of General Practice.* London: Routledge and Kegan Paul.

Cartwright, A., and Anderson, R. 1981. *General Practice Revisited: A Study of Patients and their Doctors.* London: Tavistock.

Cleary, P., Mechanic, D., and Weiss, N. 1981. "The effect of interviewer characteristics on responses to a mental health interview." *Journal of Health and Social Behavior* 22:183-93.

Davis, F. 1963. *Passage Through Crisis: Polio Victims and their Families.* Indianapolis: Bobbs-Merrill.

Dohrenwend, B.S., and Dohrenwend, B.P. (eds). 1974. *Stressful Life Events: Their Nature and Effects.* New York: John Wiley.

_____ (eds). 1981. *Stressful Life Events and their Contexts.* New Brunswick, NJ: Rutgers University Press.

Feldman, J.J. 1960. "The Household Morbidity Interview Survey as a technique for the collection of morbidity data." *Journal of Chronic Diseases* 11:535-57.

Fienberg, S.E., Loftus, E.F., and Tanor, J.L. 1985. "Cognitive aspects of health survey methodology: An overview." *The Milbank Quarterly* 63:547-64.

Goffman, E. 1961. *Asylums: Essays on the Social Situation of Mental Patients and Other Inmates.* Garden City, NY: Anchor Books.

Gortmaker, S.L., Eckenrode, J., and Gore, S. 1982. "Stress and the utilization of health services: A time series and cross-sectional analysis." *Journal of Health and Social Behavior* 23:25-38.

Hansell, S., Mechanic, D., and Brondolo, E. 1986. "Introspectiveness and adolescent development." *Journal of Youth and Adolescence* 15:115-32.

Holmes, T.H., and Rahe, R.H. 1967. "The Social Readjustment Scale." *Journal of Psychosomatic Research* 11:213-18.

Katschnig, H. 1986. "Measuring life stress—A comparison of the checklist and the panel technique." In Katschnig, H. (ed.), *Life Events and Psychiatric Disorders: Controversial Issues.* Cambridge: Cambridge University Press, 74-106.

Lazarsfeld, P. 1959. "Problems in methodology." In Merton, R., Broom, L., and Cottrell, L.S., Jr., (eds.), *Sociology Today: Problems and Prospects.* New York: Basic Books, 39-78.

Leventhal, H., Meyer, D., and Nerenz, D. 1980. "The common-sense representation of illness danger." In Rachman, S. (ed.), *Medical Psychology* 2. New York: Pergamon, 7-30.

Leventhal, H., Prohaska, T.R., and Hirschman, R.S. 1985. "Preventive health behavior across the life span." In Rosen, J.C., and Solomon, L.J. (eds.), *Prevention in Health Psychology.* Hanover, NH: University Press of New England, 191-235.

Lieberson, S. 1985. *Making it Count: The Improvement of Social Research and Theory*. Berkeley: University of California Press.

Linn, L.S. 1968a. "The mental hospital from the patient perspective." *Psychiatry* 31:213–23.

_____. 1968b. *The Mental Hospital in the Patient's Phenomenal World*. Ph.D. diss. University of Wisconsin, Madison.

Marquis, K.H., and Cannel, C.F. 1971. "Effects of some experimental interviewing techniques on reporting in the Health Interview Survey." *Vital and Health Statistics*, ser. 2, no. 41. Rockville, MD: National Center for Health Statistics.

Mechanic, D. 1989. *Mental Health and Social Policy*, 3d ed. Englewood Cliffs, NJ: Prentice-Hall.

_____. 1986. "Illness behavior: An overview." In McHugh, S., and Vallis, T.M. (eds.), *Illness Behavior: A Multidisciplinary Model*. New York: Plenum Press, 101–08.

_____. 1983. "Adolescent health and illness behavior: Review of the literature and a new hypothesis for the study of stress." *Journal of Human Stress* 9:4–13.

_____. 1980. " The experience and reporting of common physical complaints." *Journal of Health and Social Behavior* 21:597–608.

_____. 1979a. "Correlates of physician utilization: Why do major multivariate studies of physician utilization find trivial psychosocial effects." *Journal of Health and Social Behavior* 20:387–96.

_____. 1979b. "Development of psychological distress among young adults." *Archives of General Psychiatry* 36:1233–39.

_____. 1978a. *Medical Sociology*, 2d ed. New York: Free Press.

_____. 1978b. *Students Under Stress: A Study in the Social Psychology of Adaption*. Reissued with new introduction. Madison: University of Wisconsin Press.

_____. 1975. "Sociocultural and social-psychological factors affecting personal responses to psychological disorder." *Journal of Health and Social Behavior* 16:393–404.

_____. 1970. "Correlates of frustration among British general practitioners." *Journal of Health and Social Behavior* 11:87–104.

Mechanic, D., and Newton, M. 1965. "Some problems in the analysis of morbidity data." *Journal of Chronic Diseases* 18:569–80.

Nisbett, R.E., and Wilson, T.D. 1970. "Telling more than we can know: Verbal reports of mental processes." *Psychological Review* 84:231–59.

Roghmann, K.J., and Haggerty, R.J. 1972. "The diary as a research instrument in the study of health and illness behavior: Experiences with a random sample of young families." *Medical Care* 10:143–63.

Singer, B., and Marini, M.M. 1987. "Advancing social research: An essay based on Stanley Lieberson's *Making it Count*." In Clogg, C.C. (ed.), *Sociological Methodology*, vol. 17, 373–91. San Francisco: Jossey-Bass.

Stunkard, A., Foster, G., Glassman, J., and Rosato, E. 1985. "Retrospective exaggeration of symptoms: Vomiting after gastric surgery for obesity." *Psychosomatic Medicine* 47:150–55.

Tversky, A., and Kahneman, D. 1974. "Judgment under uncertainty: Heuristics and biases." *Science* 185:1124–31.

Verbrugge, L.M. 1985. "Triggers of symptoms and health care." *Social Science and Medicine* 20:855–70.

———. 1980. "Health diaries." *Medical Care* 18:73–95.

Verbrugge, L.M., and Ascione, F.J. 1987. "Exploring the iceberg: Common symptoms and how people care for them." *Medical Care* 25:539–69.

Wadden, T.A., Stunkard, A.J., and Smoller, J.W. 1986. "Dieting and depression: A methodological study." *Journal of Consulting and Clinical Psychology* 54:869–71.

Weber, M. 1949. "Objectivity in social science and social policy. " In Shils, E., and Finch, H. (eds. and trans.), *The Methodology of the Social Sciences*. New York: Free Press, 49–112.

Weinstein, Raymond M. 1983. "Labeling theory and the attitudes of mental patients." *Journal of Health and Social Behavior* 24:70–84.

———. 1979. "Patient attitudes toward mental hospitalization: A review of quantitative research." *Journal of Health and Social Behavior* 20:237–58.

Appendix B

The Role of Sociology in Health Affairs

More than a century ago, Rudolf Virchow noted that medicine is in essence a social science, and politics nothing more than medicine on a larger scale. Virchow, and many others over the past two centuries, saw the extent to which disease and epidemics derived from the material conditions of living and the social stratification of society. An enormous body of research and analysis have confirmed this observation in more recent years in relation to mortality as a whole and to a wide range of diseases and disabilities. Two important government reports in the 1980s in England (the Black Report) and in the United States (Report of the Secretary's Task Force on Black and Minority Health) reviewed the impressive evidence of the effects of socioeconomic status and racial and ethnic differences on health and longevity (Black et al. 1982; Secretary's Task Force 1985). These reports, unfortunately, were met with disfavor or embarrassment by the national administrations in the United States and England, who did little to disseminate them.

The fortunes of sociology, as well as the other social sciences, are linked with the prevailing attitudes, values, and politics of the time. While the discipline developed an institutional base at the beginning of the century, substantial growth only occurred with the rapid expansion of higher education following World War II, and postwar growth in government support for research (Bloom 1986). Membership in the national professional association was never much over 1,000 before the war, but grew rapidly after 1945, exceeding 14,000 members by 1970. Sociology and the other social sciences suffered setbacks in the 1980s, substantially as a consequence of hostility by a conservative federal administration, and the general population's shifting concerns toward personal priorities.

Sociology in Context

Sociologists played a useful role in the World War II effort exemplified by Samuel Stouffer's Research Branch of the Army's Information and Education Division, and the publication of the *American Soldier* (Stouffer et al. 1949). Yet, the social sciences were excluded when the National Science Foundation was initially established in 1946. Nevertheless, the social research activities initiated throughout government during the war became firmly established and grew in importance in subsequent decades (Lazerfield, Sewell, and Wilensky 1967). Government was less interested in basic science, however, and more in the use of social science methods—particularly the social survey and scientific sampling to answer government's informational needs. While a wide range of methodologies were introduced and found useful, including content analysis, focused interviewing, and randomized social experiments, the large-scale national survey became the launching pad for a wide array of continuing social inquiries.

With the passage in 1956 of the National Health Survey Act, which supported the establishment of the Household Interview Survey, government became involved in ongoing monitoring of the nation's health and in administering the most sophisticated and comprehensive health data collection found anywhere in the world. The range of continuing and special surveys on health care provides much of the information that allows us to assess health status and progress in relation to national objectives (National Center for Health Statistics 1989). In the National Center for Health Statistics and many other agencies of our government, sociologists and other social scientists oversee the design, implementation, analysis, and dissemination of the results of surveys on almost every aspect of our population, economy and social system.

Mental Health Roots

Sociologists worked on health issues throughout the century, but medical sociology as an institutionalized specialty first developed a strong educational infrastructure in the 1950s and 1960s, largely with the support of the National Institute of Mental Health (NIMH). Unlike the National Institute of Health (NIH), at that time NIMH saw the social and behavioral sciences as central to the development of its mission. Thus, the agency broadly invested in fellowships and training programs in sociology, psychology, and anthropology. In the 1950s and 1960s, most medical sociology was focused on mental health issues and contributed many of the concepts and much of the research that helped transform mental health services in the United States from a hospital to a community endeavor. It was the NIMH that supported studies in psychiatric epidemiology, stress and coping, public attitudes and stigma, labeling processes, the course of disability, and the study of hospitals. In those years, the emphasis was on mental health broadly conceived, and NIMH contributed importantly to the development of social and behavioral research, including the development of methodologies and analytic techniques. Under pressure during the Reagan years, NIMH very much narrowed its training and research support to focus more specifically on the mentally ill population, in contrast to broader mental health concerns.

By the 1980s, however, many of the NIH institutes recognized the importance of social and behavioral research for their missions, and helped compensate for NIMH's more narrow emphasis. The National Institute on Aging, with its broad agenda of studying developmental change across the life cycle, did much to promote improved methodology and high-quality data, and to support substantive research across a wide range of issues affecting health, function, and well-being. Similarly, the National Institute of Child Health and Human Development supported much sociological effort in the area of population research. While the heart, cancer, and other institutes were more narrowly focused, they increasingly supported epidemiological and behavioral research relevant to their categorical missions. The heart institute was particularly instrumental in developing the field of behavioral medicine.

Some Contributions of Medical Sociology

Medical sociological endeavors tend to follow two streams: sociology *in* medicine and sociology *of* medicine (Straus 1957). In the former, sociologists work as applied investigators or technicians, seeking to answer questions of interest to their sponsors, whether government agencies, foundations, hospitals, or medical schools. Depending on the ingenuity of the researcher, such work can make broader contributions than the particular task may suggest, but the emphasis is on information and application. This role is familiar, encompassing those who design and execute health surveys and who study such varied topics as access to care, use of services, satisfaction, risk factors in disease, health status determinants, and many more.

Sociology *of* medicine, in contrast, focuses on testing sociological hypotheses using medicine as an arena for studying basic issues in social stratification, power and influence, social organization, socialization, and the broad context of social values. Work within this tradition explores such themes as how physicians control the work of other health occupations; how lower social status and gender affect health interactions; and how political and economic interests influence the structure of care, reimbursement, and the uses of technology. At the organizational level, such studies commonly contrast rhetoric with reality, seeking to identify the motivations, incentives, and group interests that result in departures from public declarations and stated goals (Mechanic 1978; Freeman and Levine 1989; Waitzkin 1983; Freidson 1970a). Medical sociology has little theory of its own, depending on its parent discipline for its broader perspectives. Thus, the major points of emphasis that define sociology in general help focus the way generic questions about health and medicine are formulated.

Medical Education

Medical sociology, for example, has had long involvement in the study of medical education, dating from the 1950s. Educators sought assistance from sociologists in improving curricula and in understanding better how to structure education to deal with the stresses of training, reduce unethical behavior, improve selection processes, and induce more thoughtful inquiring behavior on the part of physicians in training—in short, how to transform students into better medical professionals. Many sociologists sharing these goals with medical educators did excellent studies on such issues as coping with uncertainty, specialty selection, factors affecting professional socialization, and the like (Merton et al. 1957; Fox 1988; Mumford 1970).

Other studies, however, examined medical education in terms of its values and contradictions. They focused on the incompatibility between educational rhetoric and the behavior of the faculty; they described the economic and prestige incentives that deterred faculty from their professed goals and values; and they viewed some of the less commen-

dable behavior of medical students as adaptive to many of the contradictory challenges and incentives to which they were exposed (Becker et al.
1961; Bloom 1971; Light 1983). They questioned whether the ethical
problem was simply a matter of more careful selection to avoid a few
"bad apples" as the physicians often saw the issue, the lack of a course
in ethics, or the result of fundamental problems concerning the incentives
and rewards within medicine. In short, they saw the problem not as one
of simple remedies. In addition, critics of medical education were less
impressed by the claims and status of the profession. While those closer
to medicine might think of medical education in terms of *The Student
Physician*, those less impressed thought of them more as *Boys in White*
(Merton et al. 1957; Becker et al. 1961).

Medical Sociology and Physicians

Work in medical sociology, more closely tied to disciplinary interests,
finds less acceptance among physicians and administrators because it
looks at issues of health and medicine from the outside, commonly
operating on premises that reject basic assumptions of the profession.
Thus, in response to one study that described the deceptions used by
house officers under pressure from their medical chief to gain autopsy
permissions (Duff and Hollingshead 1968; Ingelfinger 1968), one very
prominent physician lamented the preoccupation with "learning in its
most ghoulish aspects" and warned that it just opened "new veins of
muck for those who make it their business to rake the medical profession." An eminent physician, stung by a highly critical study of his
service, lamented that 'the authors' combination of smugness and naiveté
is hard to bear by someone who has been dealing with the realities"
(Beeson 1968; Mechanic 1974). This is just one of many instances in
which sociology from the outside was hard to take by those being studied.

Robert Petersdorf and Alvin Feinstein, in commenting on the field,
noted that such work "has been a troublesome domain for many
clinicians, who believe their distinctive concerns for individual people
are lost in collectivist beliefs about society, and whose generally conservative political views have clashed with the strongly liberal, often radical
positions of many sociologists" (Petersdorf and Feinstein 1981). It seems
clear that these commentators—and probably most of their colleagues—
prefer a sociology that is adjunct to medical activity and accepting of its

basic premises. Such a sociology would simply be a servant to medicine, not fulfilling its larger responsibility to understand medicine as a social, political, and legal endeavor; to challenge its curative and technological imperatives; to examine equity of care in relation to class, race, gender, age, character of illness, and geographic area; and to study the appropriate goals and objectives for health care in the context of an aging society with an illness trajectory dominated by chronic disease (Mechanic 1978; Aiken and Mechanic 1986; Mechanic 1983; Freeman and Levine 1989; Waitzkin 1983; Freidson 1970a, 1970b; Starr 1982).

Although the critical perspective accounts for only a part of sociological effort, it is an indispensable component. This is not to argue that such analyses are not occasionally overstated or that their failure to show understanding for the constraints under which health professionals and policymakers work sometimes undermines receptivity of the audience. Perhaps most grating to the practitioner is a tendency to view necessary restructuring less in terms of small adjustments and more in terms of major changes that, if not politically repugnant, may seem far-fetched or impractical (Alford 1975). Yet such work, and the perspectives underlying it, has been enriching and over time has been accepted as part of conventional wisdom.

Consider some of the research concerns of medical sociologists that were unpopular among many physicians. Sociologists have for decades studied organized forms of group practice, including health maintenance organizations (HMOs), making efforts to understand how alternative organization and payment arrangements affected access to and use of care and costs. Researchers have inquired how patients' social class, race, gender, and geography affect the quality of communication with health professionals and access to specialized care and how interaction and communication processes relate to adherence with medical advice, patient satisfaction, and issues of equity. Seemingly esoteric concerns of sociology have now become commonplace, such as the rights of patients in human experimentation, choices in pregnancy and childbirth, the right to be informed about the nature of one's treatment, protection against the use of medicine for social control purposes, the excessive uses of medical technology, the importance of primary care, the role of social behavior in disease and disability, and the potentials of prevention (Mechanic 1978; Freeman and Levine 1989).

Disability as an Example

Because the scope of sociology is so broad, it is more useful to convey how sociologists think than to attempt to summarize the range of their concerns. The area of disability and rehabilitation offers one important example. From the early work of Talcott Parsons, it was clear that sickness and disability were, in part, social role definitions evolving from a system of expectations and social relationships (Parsons 1951). Expectations are seen as powerful influences in society, conditioning not only what is permitted but also the human possibilities of adaptation. Social norms and social arrangements commonly result in the unnecessary exclusion of persons with disabilities from many social settings and often indirectly undermines their subsequent motivations and efforts.

Sociologists have often noted that the social definition of a chronic disease or impairment and the processes of adaptation that relate to it shape future opportunities and constraints. In such instances as myocardial infarction, spinal injury, loss of hearing or sight, and other chronic disease and impairment, persons with comparable conditions adapt in varying ways to varying degrees. Whether the condition becomes the core of the person's identity and totally incapacitates function or whether it is more peripheral depends not only on personality and motivation but also on social arrangements and public attitudes. Whether a person with an impairment becomes disabled thus depends in large part on how rehabilitation efforts are organized and the extent to which physical access, attitudes, and social reactions make jobs, recreation, and other forms of social participation feasible. Such thinking is the basis of the Americans with Disabilities Act, supported by a strong bipartisan coalition. These views are only now becoming commonplace. Yet, their foundation and philosophy have been developing for decades as a result of studies that established the deleterious ways in which people with disabilities were socially defined and dealt with (Nagi 1969; Scott 1969; Davis 1963).

The Retrenchment of the 1980s

By the 1980s, the social sciences had become a fundamental part of how we think about societal affairs; their influences are seen pervasively in the mass media, education, government, business, and health affairs.

Having a social science perspective is in some degree synonymous with being an educated and informed person. No educated person can be wholly ignorant of the role in American life of polling and surveys, of the influences of incentives on motivation and behavior, and of the importance of organization in accomplishing our objectives. Much of social science appears obvious once we assimilate the ideas into our views of the world.

Ironically, in the 1980s social science came under sustained attack by conservatives who associated these disciplines with social policies and economic theories that were critical of capitalism and extolled the welfare state (Gilder 1981; Murray 1984). Although social scientists could be found on all sides of the intellectual debate on the role of capitalism and the impact of welfare policies, conservatives perceived social scientists and their tendency to prefer government intervention in the marketplace and in many institutional spheres as "liberal." While most of social science research was peripheral to these philosophical issues, and much investigation was apolitical in its focus and concerns, sustained efforts were made to reduce research support for these disciplines. In the early Reagan years, social research at the National Science Foundation was almost eliminated, and funding for broad social inquiry at NIMH and other federal agencies was substantially constrained.

The attack on social science was coincident with efforts to reduce government programs and with an ideology that attributed the problems of welfare to the social programs of the 1960s. The evidence is that government policies in the 1980s were unkind to the poor and disabled, and especially to children (Ellwood 1988). In the period 1976 to 1987, real value of Aid to Families with Dependent Children (AFDC) benefits per family decreased by 30 to 50 percent. Between 1976 and 1984, the number of Americans in poverty increased from 25 to 34 million. By 1985, one in four children in America lived in female-headed families; more than half the children in such families are poor. Twenty percent of all children in our nation live in poverty (Bane and Ellwood 1989). Access to health care also has decreased. As many as 37 million people are uninsured, and many more are underinsured. Persons with serious chronic problems, such as the seriously mentally ill and those with chemical addictions, are greatly neglected, and the number of homeless persons has increased with the loss of low-income housing stock. Aware of a lack of sympathy with Reagan's social welfare policies, conservative officials—particularly in the first Reagan term—substantially cut funding for basic inquiry and training in the social sciences, and careers in these areas became less attractive not only economically but also in relation to the new social environment.

In the 1950s and 1960s, the social sciences had been linked with optimistic conceptions of the malleability of human nature and strong orientations to social reform. Supported by an ethos of social activism, university enrollments in sociology and other social sciences had accelerated. Social scientists became involved in public affairs and had important roles in the evolution of thinking underlying many of the social programs of the 1960s. By the 1970s the country's mood had changed and social interventions were seen increasingly in the context of failure and the costs of good intentions (Morris 1980). With few available positions in universities and little research funding, graduates could anticipate a constrained job market and difficult careers. Also, with growing emphasis on personal economic success, students refocused on business and the professions. A variety of conditions contributed to the retrenchment of sociology, including the economy and the fragmentation of the discipline itself, but the shift of emphasis to marketplace solutions in public policy and the hostility to social science added to pessimism and discouragement.

Medical Sociology and Medical Economics

Both sociology and economics were affected by the conservative attacks of the 1980s, but economics responded more resiliently. Sociologists are much more actively engaged in collecting primary data, but the high cost and cutbacks in funding made this difficult. Social scientists using secondary data sources had a distinct advantage, a fact favoring economists and quantitatively oriented sociologists. Also, unlike sociology, economics had a broader base of support through employment in the private sector. Most sociologists outside of academia were in government agencies, and this was not an exciting time to be a bureaucrat. Economics was alone in retaining a core paradigm that was widely held whatever the individual differences among economists, while the other social sciences became increasingly specialized and fragmented. Unlike earlier periods, there was no longer any single theoretical paradigm that was commonly shared, and it became more difficult to identify common perspectives and assumptions that defined the work of the disciplines. In sociology, for example, existing differences in theoretical perspectives, in adherence to quantitative and qualitative methods, in theoretical versus applied concerns, and in specific areas of interest became accentuated. It has become increasingly difficult to identify the common core that defines a sociologist, and definition occurs more typically by methodological approach than by a common theory. Research as it applies to health and health policy shares these characteristics.

In the area of scholarship on health and health affairs, attention in the 1980s has focused substantially on issues of financing, reimbursement, and cost-containment mechanisms. While in the 1960s and 1970s, access and quality were equal partners in the access/cost/quality triad, in the decade of the 1980s they became secondary to cost. Consistent with national and state policy concerns with mounting health care costs, pressures on public financing, and the pragmatic politics that accompanied these concerns, research questions about social justice and humanistic concerns were not high on the national agenda; nor were such previous common concerns as patient and provider satisfaction, the quality of provider/patient relationships, collaborative relationships among the health professions, and many more.

The political and social trends of the 1980s, and the growing dependence on secondary data, reinforced an already clear preference for addressing narrow research questions amenable to sophisticated quantitative methods and modeling techniques. Funded research in health emphasized cost issues, and the health research agenda became more restricted than it had been in previous decades. Strong interest in information on social problems did persist, but even our data systems suffered erosion due to budget constraints and a lack of receptivity to what was going to be bad news. The political environment was particularly inhospitable to analyses and interpretations that viewed problems of the poor, the homeless, the disabled, and the uninsured more as products of our social arrangements and politics than as the vulnerabilities, qualities, and choices of those affected. Moreover, in certain areas of American life, even factual investigation remains taboo. The current stalemate in gaining approval for a scientific survey of sexual behavior—a survey of vital importance for tracking the AIDS epidemic and planning AIDS prevention programs—suggests the complex ways in which values shape even attitudes about collection of information.

Shift from Sociology to Economics

It is not difficult to appreciate, thus, why the center of gravity in research on health research has shifted to the economic sciences. Economists bring to the area a widely shared and powerful conception of rational choice based on the dynamics of supply and demand. To many economists, purchasing health care is fundamentally no different than purchasing carrots or cameras, and many of the uncertainties or imperfections of medical care markets can be accounted for by "information costs," the residual category of economic analysis that seemingly explains away many of the core concerns of the other social sciences.

Even when supply and demand analysis proves deficient, as in efforts to explain surgical fees or the consequences of the increasing supply of professionals, the presence of an agreed-upon paradigm, when the other social sciences are each floundering to identify what their practitioners share in common, gives economics a strong advantage. Economists also bring sophisticated econometric techniques and models to their work, tools highly adaptable to the questions on which governments and policy focus. While economists come in all political persuasions, the paradigmatic orientation of most American economists is inherently conservative, and most are unlikely to challenge the deeper assumptions of public policy orientations. Health economics still remains a relatively new player, not yet fully established in its own basic discipline, which values theory and method far more than the applied concerns to which health economists apply themselves. But the compatibility between economic theory and method and the issues that most concern health policymakers has put health economics in the ascendancy. These factors increasingly dominate the way health questions are being framed.

Unlike economics, which is highly focused, medical sociology covers an extraordinarily broad range of issues in social epidemiology, health care organization, patient/practitioner interactions, illness behavior, patient expectations and responses, the course of chronic disease, the organization of the health professions, and many more. The medical sociology section of the American Sociological Association had more than 1,100 members in 1987—almost 10 percent of its total membership.

Because of the dispersion of efforts and the diversity of quantitative and qualitative methods medical sociologists use, they are often not easily distinguished from social epidemiologists, survey and evaluation researchers, and other researchers in public health and health services. While many medical sociologists are directly concerned with health policy issues, much of everyday activity involves gathering basic health status information, studying the social causes of illness and disability and their course, and examining factors associated with positive health status and behavior.

The Future of Medical Sociology

Early publications from the RAND Health Insurance Experiment on the effects of copayment on ambulatory care reinforced interest in a market approach to health care (Newhouse et al. 1981). Later analyses that have received considerably less attention show that copayment had a diffuse effect on the use of services affecting appropriate and efficacious care and less efficacious care equally (Lohr et al. 1986). In short, contrary to much opinion and rhetoric, copayment was not selective in what services it reduced. Other analyses showed larger effects of copayment on the sick poor than on the affluent and showed that medical care had little impact on a broad array of outcome measures (Brook et al. 1983). In short, the Health Insurance Experiment and many of the studies that followed point to the extent to which the course of disease and the dynamics of the behavior of patients and health professionals are governed by noneconomic factors.

The uncontrollable costs of medical care will continue to occupy a central place on the policy agenda because of their implications for government budgets and tax demands, and their potential influence on the competitiveness of American business. But as we look ahead, it is clear that our health care system is in considerable trouble. Inequities have increased in access to care and in the quality of service, and significant proportions of our population are under- or uninsured. Encouragement of competitiveness has basically demolished our system of community rating, making it difficult for those who most need health insurance to obtain it. Tax subsidies for insurance give substantial entitlements to the most affluent, encouraging overinsurance and overuse among those who need care the least. We lack a viable strategy for organizing or paying for long-term care, despite the growing size of the elderly population and the old-old subgroup. Care for chronic illness—and particularly the stigmatized chronically mentally ill, alcohol and chemical abusers, and people with AIDS—is fragmented and in disarray. In the face of galloping medical technology, we lack standards of care and waste enormous resources through unnecessary and inappropriate procedures. Administrative costs are extraordinarily high. And, we have yet to effectively engage the tough ethical issues that biomedical advances make inevitable.

Examination of the future health care agenda makes it abundantly clear that if we didn't have a sociology of health we would now have to invent one. The influences affecting health and the provision of services are largely social, and the way we address problems of illness and care reflects our values and the arrangement of powerful interests within our social system. In a recent volume issued by the Henry J. Kaiser Family Foundation, *Pathways to Health: The Role of Social Factors*, substantial documentation is again presented illustrating the pervasive influence of socioeconomic factors on disease processes, health status, longevity, and access to medical care (Bunker et al. 1989). The integrity of our health care system requires that we address questions relating to such broad influences as well as the more technical immediate ones and that we critically examine our goals and initiatives in the light of the best scientific knowledge of the determinants of health and welfare. There is little doubt that the powerful interests in our health care system, and our political processes of decision making, create serious obstacles to fundamental change (Mechanic 1989). Nevertheless, a clear view of our goals, and the structures necessary to implement them, is an essential basis for constructive advancement.

References

Aiken, L., and Mechanic, D. 1986. *Applications of Social Sciences to Clinical Medicine and Health Policy*. New Brunswick, NJ: Rutgers University Press.
Alford, R. 1975. *Health Care Politics: Ideological and Interest Group Barriers to Reform*. Chicago: University of Chicago Press.
Bane, M.J., and Ellwood, D.T. 1989. "One-fifth of the nation's children: Why are they poor?" *Science* 245:1047–53
Becker, H., Geer, B., Hughes, E.C., and Strauss, A.M. 1961. *Boys in White: Student Culture in the Medical School*. Chicago: University of Chicago Press

Beeson, P.B. 1968. "Special review of sickness and society." *Yale Journal of Biology and Medicine* 41:226–40.

Black. Sir D., Morris, J.N., Smith, C.S., and Townsend, P. 1982. *Inequalities in Health.* Middlesex, England: Penguin Books.

Bloom, S.W. 1986. "Institutional trends in medical sociology." *Journal of Health and Social Behavior* 27:265–76.

_____. 1971. "The medical school as a social system: A case study of faculty-student relations." *The Milbank Quarterly* 49, pt 2.

Brook, R.H., Ware, J.E., Jr., Rogers, W.H., Keeler, E.B., Davies, A.R., Donald, C.A., Goldberg, G.A., Lohr, K.N., Masthay, P.C., and Newhouse, J.P. 1983. "Does free care improve adults' health? Results from a randomized controlled trial." *New England Journal of Medicine* 309:1426–32.

Bunker, J.P., Gomby, D.S., and Kehrer, B.H. (eds.). 1989. *Pathways to Health: The Role of Social Factors.* Menlo Park, CA: Henry J. Kaiser Family Foundation.

Davis, F. 1963. *Passage Through Crisis.* Indianapolis: Bobbs-Merrill.

Duff, R.S., and Hollingshead, A.B. 1968. *Sickness and Society.* New York: Harper and Row.

Ellwood, D.T. 1988. *Poor Support: Poverty in the American Family.* New York: Basic Books.

Fox, R. 1988. *Essays in Medical Sociology,* 2d ed. New Brunswick, NJ: Transaction Publishers.

Freeman, H.E., and Levine, S. 1989. *Handbook of Medical Sociology,* 4th ed. Englewood Cliffs, NJ: Prentice Hall.

Freidson, E. 1970a. *Profession of Medicine.* New York: Dodd Mead.

_____. 1970b. *Professional Dominance: The Social Structure of Medical Care.* New York: Atherton.

Gilder, G. 1981. *Wealth and Poverty.* New York: Basic Books.

Ingelfinger, F.J. 1968. "The arch-hospital: An ailing monopoly." *Harper's Magazine* 237:82–87.

Institute of Medicine. 1987. *Pain and Disability: Clinical, Behavioral, and Public Policy Perspectives.* Washington, DC: National Academy Press.

Lazerfield, P.F., Sewell, W.H., and Wilensky, H.L. (eds.). 1967. *The Uses of Sociology.* New York: Basic Books.

Light, D. 1983. "Medical and nursing education: Surface behavior and deep structure." In Mechanic, D. (ed.), *Handbook of Health, Health Care, and the Health Care Professions.* New York: Free Press, 455–78.

Lohr, K.N., Brook, R.H., Kamberg, C.J., Goldberg, A., Leibowitz, A., Keesey, J., Reboussin, D., and Newhouse, J.P. 1986. *Use of Medical Care in the Rand Health Insurance Experiment: Diagnosis- and Service-Specific Analyses in a Randomized Controlled Trial.* Publication No. R–3469–HHS. Santa Monica, CA: RAND Corporation.

Mechanic, D. 1989. "Social policy, technology, and the rationing of health care." *Medical Care Review* 46:113–20.

_____. (ed.). 1983. *Handbook of Health, Health Care and the Health Professions.* New York: Free Press.

_____. 1978. *Medical Sociology,* 2d ed. New York: Free Press

_____. 1974. "Policy studies and medical-care research." *Politics, Medicine and Social Science.* New York: Wiley, 59–67.

Merton, R., Reader, G., and Kendall, P.L. (eds). 1957. *The Student Physician: Introductory Studies in the Sociology of Medical Education.* Cambridge: Harvard University Press

Morris, C. 1980. *The Cost of Good Intentions.* New York: W.W. Norton.

Mumford, E. 1970. *Interns: From Students to Physicians.* Cambridge: Harvard University Press.

Murray, C. 1984. *Losing Ground: American Social Policy, 1950–1980.* New York: Basic Books.

Nagi, S.Z. 1969. *Disability and Rehabilitation: Legal, Clinical, and Self-Concepts and Measurement.* Columbus, OH: State University Press.

National Center for Health Statistics. 1989. *Health, United States, 1988.* DHHS Pub. No. (PHS) 89-1232. Washington, DC: U.S. Government Printing Office.

Newhouse, J.P., Manning, W.G., Morris, C.N., Orr, L.L., Duan, N., Keeler, E.B., Leibowitz, A., Marquis, K.H., Marquis, M.S., Phelps, C.E., and Brook, R.H., 1981. "Some interim results from a controlled trial of cost sharing in health insurance." *New England Journal of Medicine* 305:1501-07.

Parsons, T. 1951. *The Social System.* New York: Free Press.

Petersdorf, R.G., and Feinstein, A.R. 1981. "An informal appraisal of the current status of medical sociology." In Eisenberg, L. and Kleinman, A. (eds.), *The Role of Social Science for Medicine.* Dordrecht: Reidel Publishing Co., 27-45.

Scott, R. 1969. *The Making of Blind Men: A Study of Adult Socialization.* New York: Russell Sage Foundation.

Secretary's Task Force. 1985. *Black and Minority Health.* Washington, DC: U.S. Department of Health and Human Services.

Starr, P. 1982. *The Social Transformation of American Medicine.* New York: Basic Books.

Stouffer, S.A., Lumsdaine, A.A., Lumsdaine, M.H., Williams, R.M., Smith, M.B., Janis, I.L., Steu, S.A., and Cottrell, L.S. (eds.). 1949. *The American Soldier, Studies in Social Psychology of World War II,* 4 vols. Princeton: Princeton University Press.

Straus, R. 1957. "The nature and status of medical sociology." *American Sociological Review* 22: 200-4.

Waitzkin, H. 1983. *The Second Sickness: Contradictions of Capitalist Health Care.* New York: Free Press.

Index